MW00637036

HEALING TONICS, JUICES, AND SMOOTHIES

Skyhorse Publishing books may be purchased in bulk at special discounts for sales promotion, corporate gifts, fund-raising, or educational purposes. Special editions can also be created to specifications. For details, contact the Special Sales Department, Skyhorse Publishing, 307 West 36th Street, 11th Floor, New York, NY 10018 or info@skyhorsepublishing.com.

Skyhorse® and Skyhorse Publishing® are registered trademarks of Skyhorse Publishing, Inc.®, a Delaware corporation.

Visit our website at www.skyhorsepublishing.com.

10 9 8 7 6 5

Library of Congress Cataloging-in-Publication Data:

Names: Weston, Jessica Jean, author.
Title: Healing tonics, juices, and smoothies : 100+ elixirs to nurture body
   and soul / Jessica Jean Weston.
Description: New York : Skyhorse Publishing, [2017]
Identifiers: LCCN 2017004707| ISBN 9781510716292 (hardback) | ISBN
   9781510716308 (ebook)
Subjects: LCSH: Tonics (Medicinal preparations) | Beverages--Therapeutic use.
Classification: LCC RM239 .W47 2017 | DDC 613.2--dc23
LC record available at https://lccn.loc.gov/2017004707

Cover design by Jane Sheppard
Photography by Wyatt Andrews
Author photo by Jacob Roberts

Print ISBN: 978-1-5107-1629-2
Ebook ISBN: 978-1-5107-1630-8

Printed in China

DISCLAIMER: This book is not meant to be used to diagnose or treat any medical conditions. Consult your physician for diagnosis or treatment of any medical conditions. Always consult a physician before starting a new diet or wellness program.

HEALING TONICS, JUICES, AND SMOOTHIES

100+ ELIXIRS TO NURTURE BODY AND SOUL

JESSICA JEAN WESTON

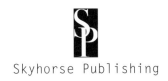

Skyhorse Publishing

TABLE OF CONTENTS

EQUIPMENT   226

SOURCING   230

CUSTOM SUPERFOOD ADD-ON GUIDE   232

NUT + SEED SOAKING GUIDE   233

INGREDIENT GLOSSARY   234

RESOURCES   251

ACKNOWLEDGMENTS   253

ABOUT THE AUTHOR   255

INDEX   256

INTRODUCTION

tonic: a medicinal substance taken to give a feeling of vigor or well-being

Happy health, wellness warrior! I am extremely excited to share these simple recipes for vibrant health with you in *Healing Tonics, Juices, and Smoothies.* Jumping into the deep end of the vast world of health food can be daunting and almost paralyzing, depending on your point of entry, and I would like to take this moment to give you a big high-five for picking up and reading this book! That is a huge step toward taking charge of your life. While I won't claim that owning this book and making these recipes will be a cure-all, they are sure to help increase your vitality and broaden your imagination (and flavor palate) of what healthy beverages can be.

Drinks are wonderful tools for wellness, as the majority of them are extremely simple to make (i.e., throw the ingredients into a blender or juicer and enjoy!), allowing them to become daily staples. This is also an area in the American diet where many unwanted calories are slugged down almost unknowingly. While most of the drinks in this book definitely contain calories, and you don't want to overdo it, adding them to your diet will: help to eliminate potential unhealthy beverage choices; boost your health in a myriad of ways; and be so delicious you won't know why you hadn't tried them sooner!

In this book, we'll explore the surface of the immense world of healthy beverages. Before jumping into the recipes, be sure to review some of the basic terminology that you'll encounter throughout the book, such as adaptogens and probiotics. From there we'll begin with **Herbal Teas** that can be deliciously enjoyed as they are or used as a base (substitute for hot or cold water) in other drinks for extra medicinal potency. Next on our journey we'll touch base with a few **Basic Staples**, such as Mylks, that you'll always want to have on hand. Moving on we'll jump into **Cooling Libations**, followed by **Hot Elixirs**, featuring classics such as Golden Mylk (p 59), Chaga Chai (p 67), and 'Nog (p 51), along with many other exciting concoctions.

Now that you've already taken the leap, we'll navigate the world of **Power-Packed Shots,** sure to boost your body to new heights of immunity. Since we're on the subject of healthy beverages, there is simply no way around the inclusion of two of my favorite chapters: **Invigorating Juices** and **Superfood Smoothies.** Here you'll find many classics, fun twists, and seasonal specialties:

think Wild Pine-Apple Fennel (p 105) green juice filled with wild dandelion greens you can literally walk out your back door to pick and then throw into your juicer; Funky Monkey (p 129), a protein-rich throwback to a classic combo of banana, chocolate, and (in this case) almond butter; and Caramel Apple (p 163), the ultimate happiness smoothie for cozy autumn days with crisp, crunchy, fallen leaves blanketing the ground.

In our final beverage section we'll get slightly more complex with probiotic-rich **Fanciful Ferments.** Don't let the detailed directions in this section scare you off; fermented drinks are simple, and I'll walk you through the process step by step. They are definitely worth the wait (some are ready in as little as one to two days, while others in this chapter can take up to fourteen). These brews are delicious, beautiful on your kitchen counter, and a great way to get your daily dose of probiotics.

As a bonus to the multitude of beverages, I've added in three **Nourishing Cleanses**, Raw, Candida / Alkaline, and Ayurvedic Inspired, that include raw and cooked food recipes, such as Raw Mac n' Cheeze (p 195), Seaweed Salad (p 199), Millet Croquettes (p 211), and Kitchari (p 225). The cleanses in this section will guide you on three very different experiences for hitting that occasional, much-needed reset button.

To close out our journey, I have included information on **Equipment, Sourcing, Ingredients,** Educational **Resources,** and a **Custom Superfood Add-On Guide** to further support you on your adventure.

I have my small handful of go-to drinks that I enjoy frequently, while others are more seasonal offerings or were created to satisfy particular cravings.

Whether you are a beginner or a well-versed superfoodie, I hope this book serves as a massive launchpad of learning and expansion for you to take inspiration from many of the recipes and PLAY! Get creative, try new flavor combinations, and have fun!

Cheers!

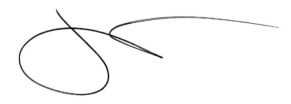

HELPFUL TERMS

ADAPTOGENS are well known in herbal medicine as natural substances, usually herbs, that help our bodies in adapting to stress and creating a balanced state.

AYURVEDA is the oldest known medical system, dating back at least 5,000 years, with origins in India's Vedic culture. It's based on the belief that a balanced body, mind, and spirit is the core to health and wellness. There are three main doshas in Ayurveda: kapha, pitta, and vata. Each individual has a different doshic makeup, which determines both physical and emotional characteristics along with treatment methods. While most people predominantly identify with one or two doshas, there is wide range of possibilities.

ELIXIR, defined as a "magical or medicinal potion," believed to extend life.

FAT is a very deceptive and usually unwelcome word in the health world, as it has been long considered physically fattening to consume fatty foods. However, it is simply an essential nutrient needed as an energy source for the body. There are different kinds of fat, some good and some bad. The sources of fat featured in this book (avocadoes, nuts, coconut oil, etc.) provide the body with healthy fatty acids, raise good cholesterol (HDL) and lower bad cholesterol (LDL). These fats have also been shown to aid in weight loss. Don't fear fat!

FERMENTATION is a process that converts sugars to acids and alcohols. Starter cultures are sometimes used, however they're not always necessary, depending on what you're making. For instance, kvass, tepache, and sauerkraut are examples of ferments that rely on the "wild" fermentation process by utilizing the natural beneficial bacteria in the ingredients, whereas kombucha and kefir require starter cultures.

GLUTEN is a mixture of proteins present in glutenous grains, such as wheat, barley, rye, and spelt.

GLUTEN-FREE diets are safe for those with celiac disease or non-celiac gluten sensitivity, as they eliminate all gluten, including foods that may be cross-contaminated because they are made in the same facility as other products that may contain gluten.

PROBIOTICS are natural substances that promote the growth of beneficial bacteria, primarily in the gut.

PROTEIN is defined as large biomolecules made up of one or more chains of amino acid residues. Due to popularized nutrition fads and misinformation, many only think of protein as something that is found in animal products. However, plants contain a vast amount of proteins as well, some more so than animal counterparts. For example, per calorie, kale contains more protein than steak. Plant-based protein is usually more bioavailable for the body to assimilate. There is also a misconceived notion that the human body needs to consume much more protein than it actually does; while this is still highly debated, there has been a great deal of research showing that most of us simply do not need as much as the daily requirements suggest.

RAW or living foods are never heated above 118 degrees F, retaining their high vibrational, nutritional structure, which is considered to be drastically decreased once cooked using high heat.

SUPERFOODS are nutrient-dense foods considered advantageous for overall well-being. They are usually consumed in smaller dosages than their edible counterparts. For example, you wouldn't eat more than a few tablespoons of cacao powder, while you could eat an entire bunch of kale.

VEGAN lifestyles do not include the use of any animal products, from food consumption to fashion. Dietarily speaking, this eliminates the consumption of animal protein, such as meat, fish, dairy, eggs, and usually bee products (such as honey, bee pollen, and propolis); some vegans or, as I've recently heard some say, "beegans," do not eat any animal protein, but do enjoy raw honey and bee products sourced from their local beekeeper.

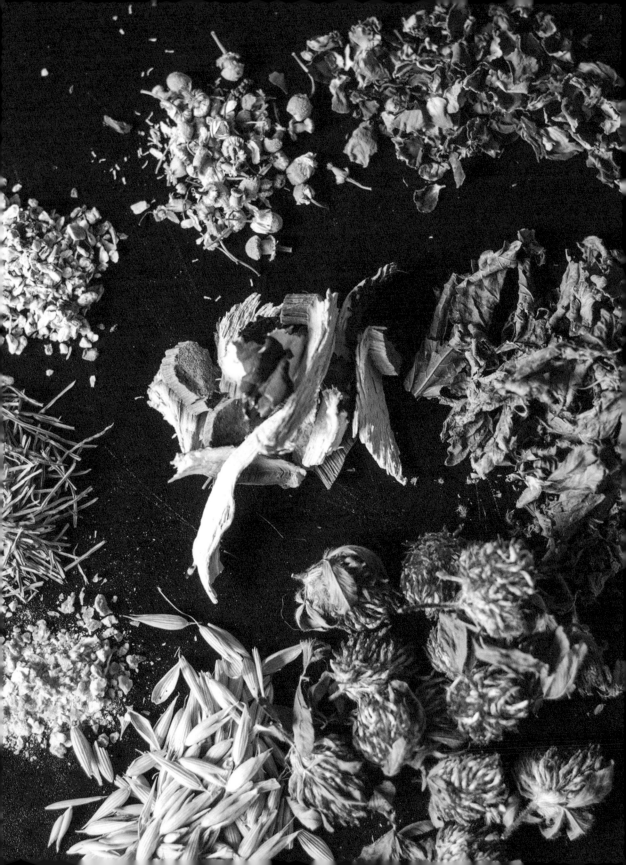

HERBAL TEAS

Herbal teas are a wonderful addition to daily life. The recipes in this chapter offer a wide range, encompassing a myriad of health benefits. Drink them as is, use these recipes as inspiration, or create as a base to blend with other recipes in this book.

When I realized that I could use medicinal teas instead of simply water when cooking or making drinks to infuse so much more medicine into my diet, my mind was officially blown, and I have rarely looked back.

While I don't always take the time to make a brew first with my busy lifestyle, it is a simple addition when you have a little extra time.

Any time a recipe calls for water, for example, in your mylks, hot elixirs, soups, cooking grains / beans, etc., you could swap it out with one of these infusions. Taste the tea first to make sure the flavor will complement the dish; some recipes will work with any tea, while others may be more particular. As a general rule of thumb, Nourishing (p 3) and Medicinal Mushroom (p 5) go with practically everything, in my mind.

TIP: I would recommend avoiding this swap out with ferments, as some herbs may affect the somewhat fragile fermentation process in a different manner than water.

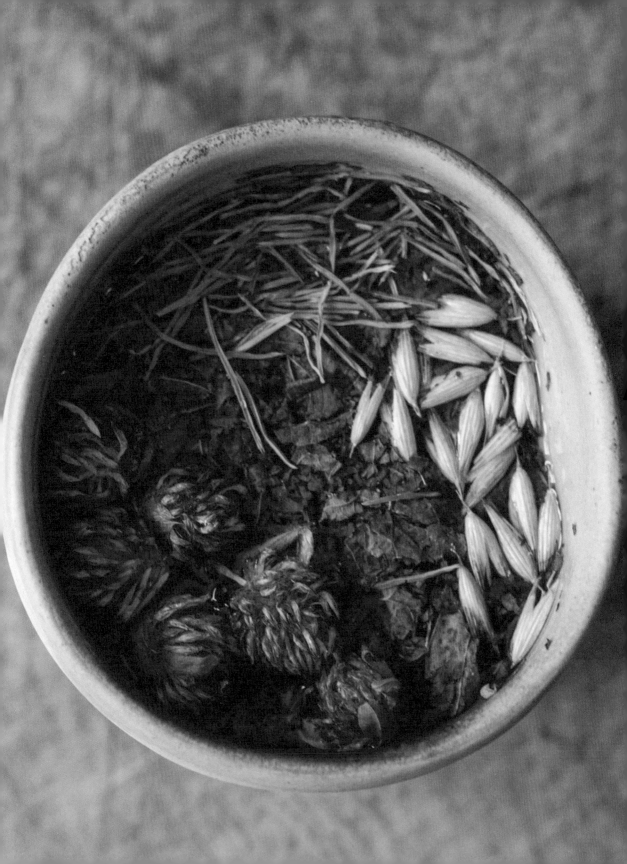

NOURISHING

Yield: 2 cups

This is one of my top two favorite teas (along with Medicinal Mushroom) for close to daily use, especially in the colder months. As its name implies, this tea is highly nourishing for the entire body and adrenal system. It's a great everyday boost to keep you going strong through shifting seasons and stressful times.

2 cups filtered water
2 tbsp dried nettle
1 tbsp horsetail
1 tbsp oat straw
2 tbsp clover

Bring the water to a boil in a teakettle. Place all the herbs in a teapot or glass jar. Once the water has boiled, pour it into the teapot over herbs, place the cover on the teapot, and let steep for at least five minutes. Strain tea to serve. Herbal teas can steep longer to release even more medicinal qualities and flavor, or add more hot water and do a second brew.

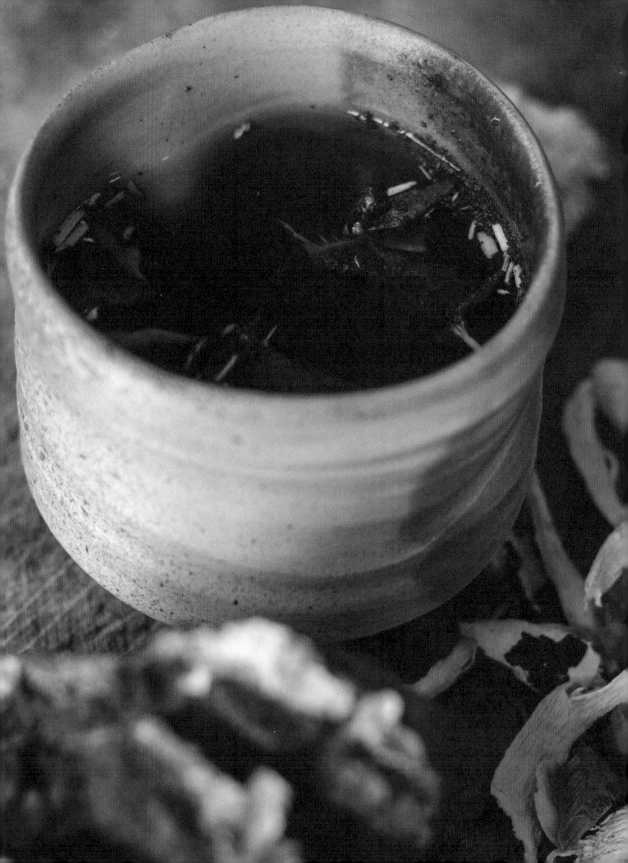

MEDICINAL MUSHROOM

Yield: 2 cups

I almost always have at least some variation of this tea in a big pot on my stovetop—often it is only chaga. These mushrooms are so potent and antibacterial / antifungal that you can leave them out (covered) and simply reheat before use. There is so much medicine in them that you can keep adding water and brewing more and more tea over a long period of time, continuing to extract as much healing goodness as possible; this is important to get out as much medicine as we can, minimize waste of these potent herbs, and use them sustainably. You should be able to easily tell by the strength of the tea if you have worn out their benefits.

2½ cups filtered water
1 tsp chaga powder
1 thin slice reishi mushroom, approximately 3 inches long
1 tbsp astragalus root

Add all ingredients to a small saucepot and brew over low heat for at least 20 minutes, until the liquid is extremely dark. Strain tea to serve. The longer these medicinal mushrooms and root brew, the more medicinal qualities will be extracted into the tea.

TIP: This makes an amazing base for soup broths and can be used to replace your water for hot drinks or when cooking grains / legumes / oatmeal.

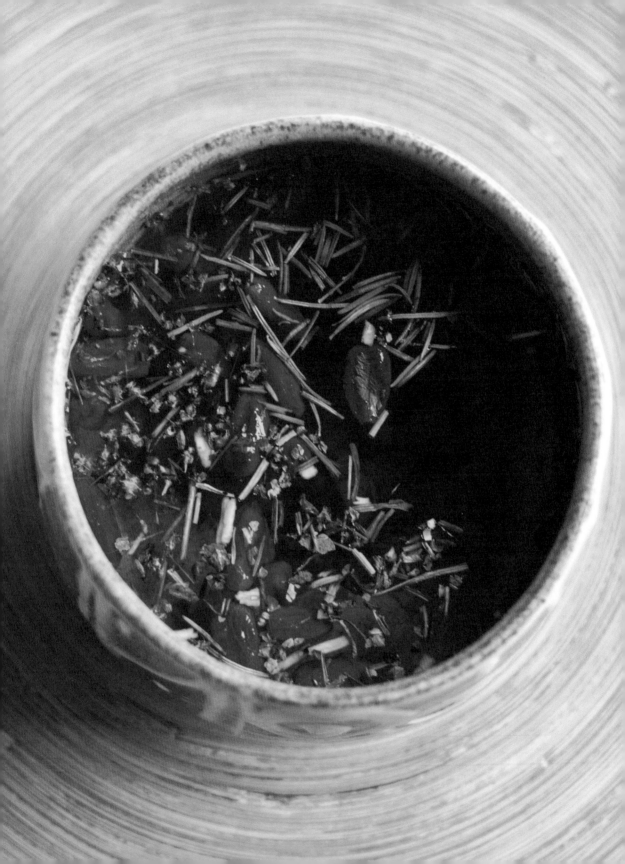

MENTAL CLARITY

Yield: 2 cups

Brew this blend when you're feeling a little foggy or need to focus on a project with super alert energy.

2 cups filtered water
1 tsp ginseng root
1 tsp gotu kola
1 tsp ashwagandha root
1 tbsp tulsi, fresh or dried
1 tsp rosemary, fresh or dried
1 tbsp goji berries

Bring the water to a boil in a teakettle. Place all the herbs in a teapot or glass jar. Once the water has boiled, pour it over the herbs, place the cover on the teapot, and let steep for at least five minutes. Strain the tea and serve. Herbal teas can steep longer to release even more medicinal qualities and flavor, or add more hot water and do a second brew.

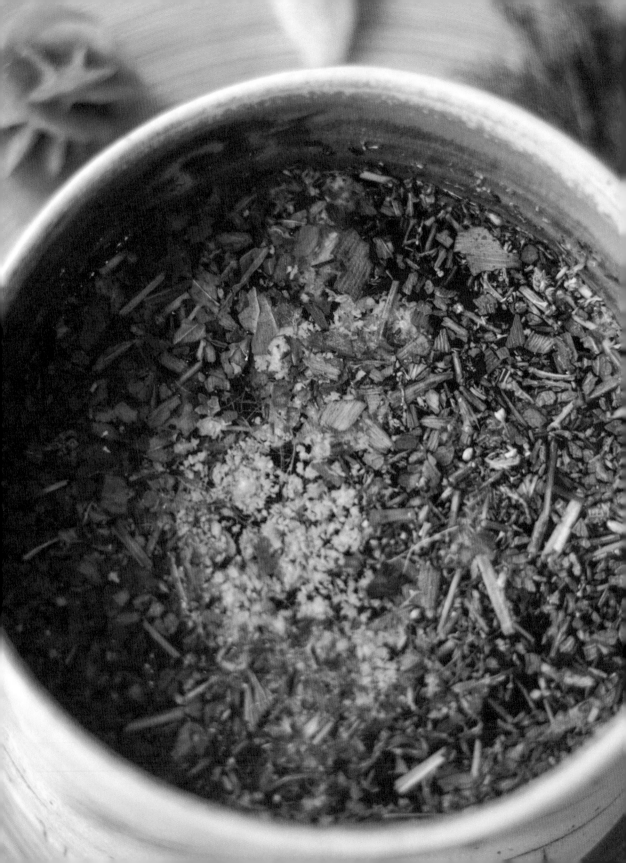

MAMA MOON

Yield: 2 cups

A loving blend to nourish and support the sacred feminine moon time. These herbs will hold space for your body and soul, relieve cramps, and aid with PMS.

2 cups filtered water
1-inch piece fresh ginger root, sliced
1 tbsp dried yarrow
2 tsp jasmine
1 tsp blue vervain
1 tsp gingko biloba
1 tsp skullcap

Bring the water to a boil in a teakettle. Place all the herbs in a teapot or glass jar. Once the water has boiled, pour it over the herbs, put the cover on the teapot, and let steep for at least five minutes. Strain tea to serve. Herbal teas can steep longer to release even more medicinal qualities and flavor, or add more hot water and do a second brew.

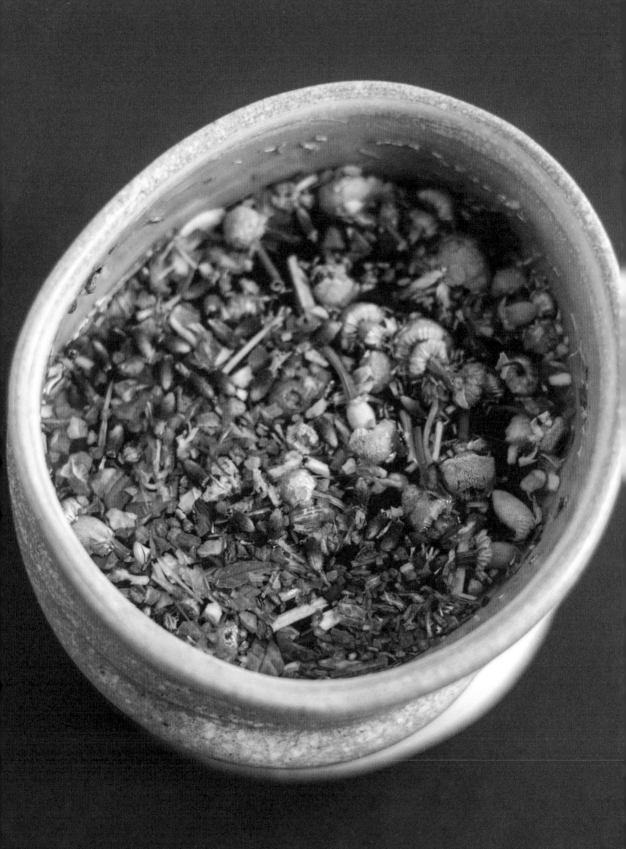

SWEET SLUMBER

Yield: 2 cups

Cozy up with this lovely floral tonic for sweet dreams and rejuvenating slumber. If you suffer from insomnia, these herbs should help support your journey toward better sleep.

2 cups filtered water
1 tsp passionflower
1 tsp blue vervain
1 tsp ashwagandha root
1 tbsp dried chamomile
1 tsp dried lavender
1 tsp skullcap

Bring water to a boil in a teakettle. Place all the herbs in a teapot or glass jar. Once the water has boiled, pour it over the herbs, put the cover on the teapot, and let steep for at least five minutes. Strain tea to serve. Herbal teas can steep longer to release even more medicinal qualities and flavor, or add more hot water and do a second brew.

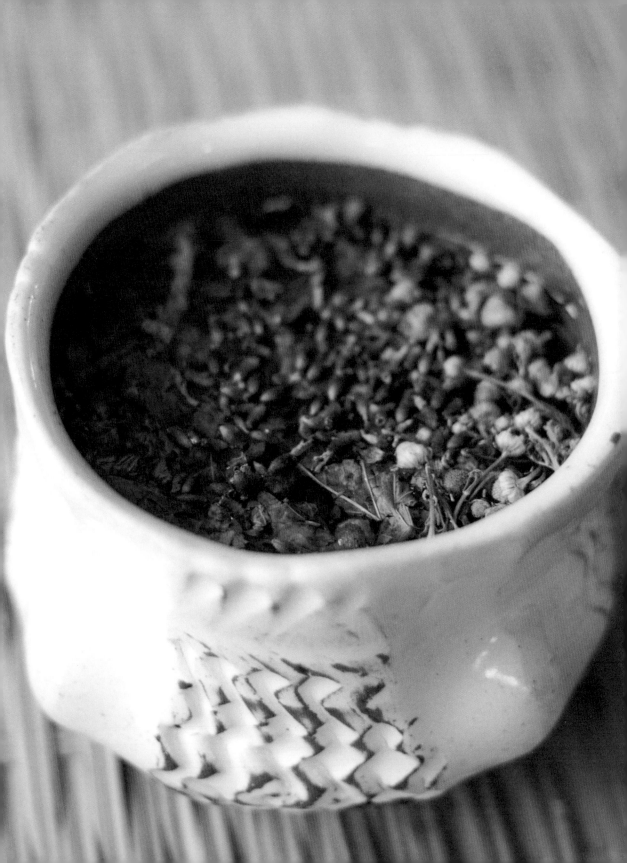

SACRED SURRENDER

Yield: 2 cups

Breathe in, breathe out. Sink into the depths of your soul . . . and then delve even further. Release. Let go. Surrender.

Sip this brew to calm the nerves and relax the mind. This tea can also be enjoyed before sleep for a restful night.

2 cups filtered water
2 tsp dried lavender
1 tbsp dried chamomile
1 tbsp dried lemon balm

Bring the water to a boil in a teakettle. Put all the herbs in a teapot or glass jar. Once the water has boiled, pour it over the herbs, place the cover on the teapot, and let steep for at least five minutes. Strain tea and serve. Herbal teas can steep longer to release even more medicinal qualities and flavor, or add more hot water and do a second brew.

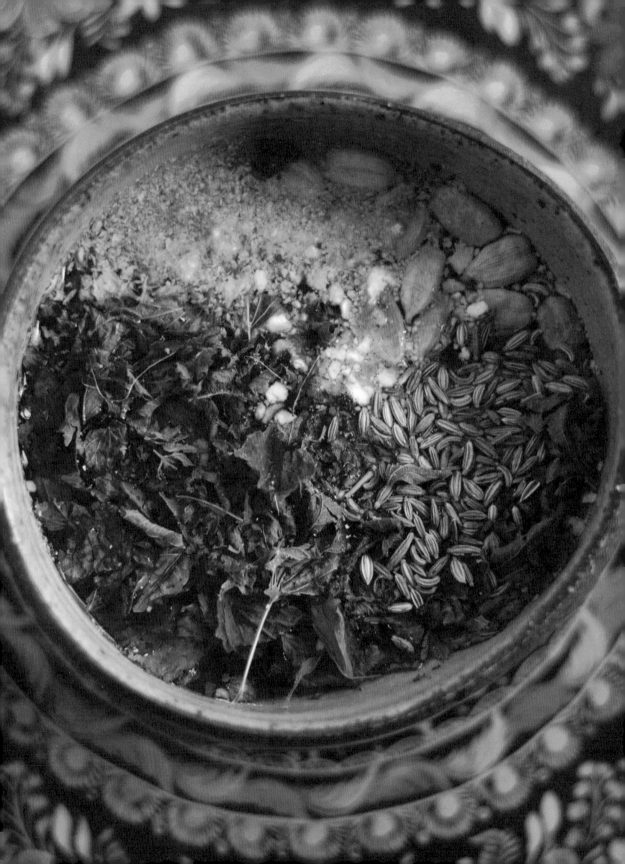

BALANCED BELLY

Yield: 2 cups

Ideal for after a meal, this digestive blend can be used to prevent or alleviate an upset stomach.

2 cups filtered water
1-inch piece fresh ginger root, sliced thin
½ tsp fennel seeds
½ tsp cardamom powder
1 tbsp dried lemon balm
1 tsp dried orange peel

Bring the water to a boil in a teakettle. Put all the herbs in a teapot or glass jar. Once the water has boiled, pour it over herbs, place the cover on the teapot, and let steep for at least five minutes. Strain tea and serve. Herbal teas can steep longer to release even more medicinal qualities and flavor, or add more hot water and do a second brew.

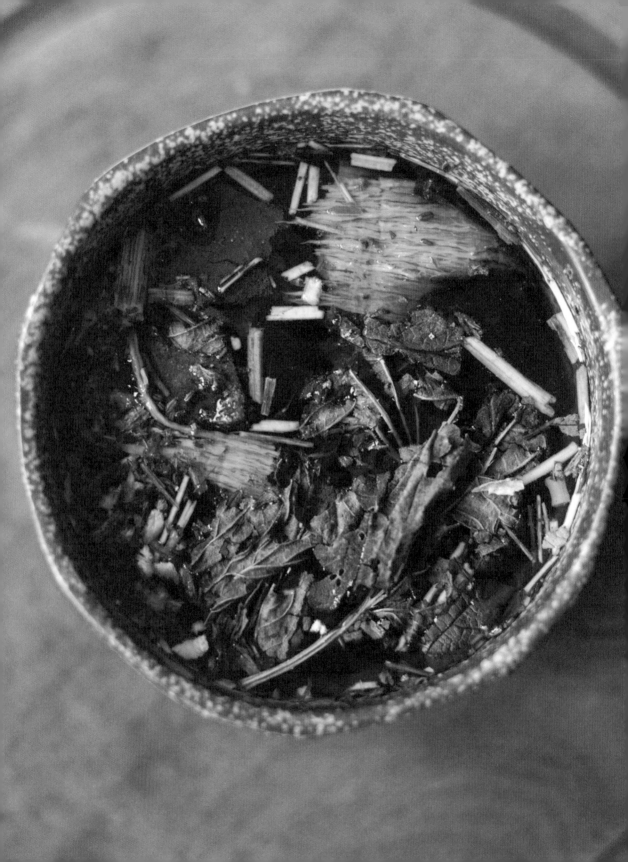

LIVER LOVER

Yield: 2 cups

The liver removes toxins from our bodies. Cleansing the liver, and therefore flushing out these toxins, can boost immunity, aid in weight loss, increase energy, and enhance overall vitality. Safely support your body in cleansing with this liver tonic. Liver Lover is a wonderful addition to any detox.

2 cups filtered water
1 tsp dandelion root
1 tsp blue vervain
1 tsp milk thistle
1 tsp burdock root
1 tsp chicory root
1 tbsp dried nettle
1 thin slice reishi mushroom, approximately 3 inches long

Bring the water to a boil in a teakettle. Place all the herbs in a teapot or glass jar. Once the water has boiled, pour it over the herbs, put the cover on the teapot, and let steep for at least five minutes. Strain tea and serve. Herbal teas can steep longer to release even more medicinal qualities and flavor, or add more hot water and do a second brew.

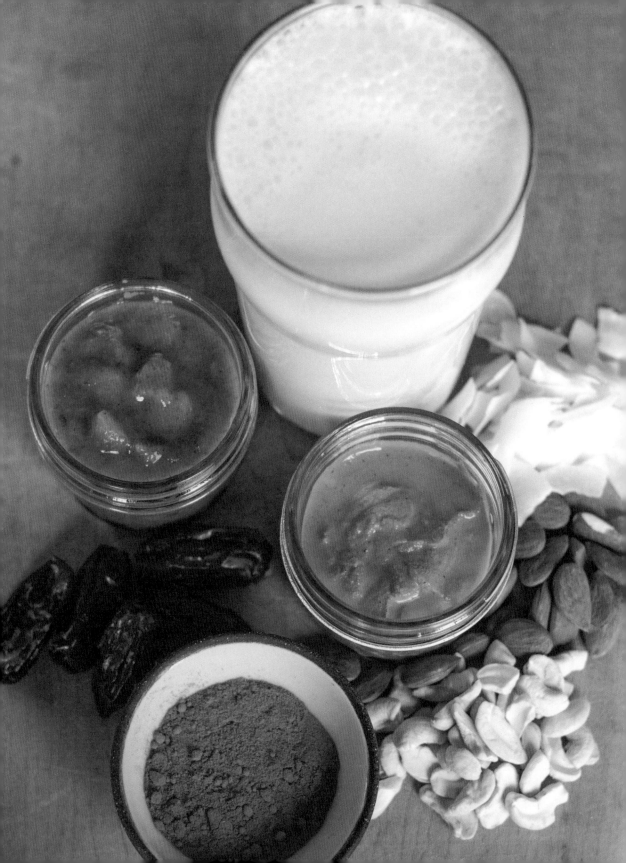

BASIC STAPLES

These three staples are extremely easy additions to spruce up any home refrigerator and have you ready to tackle all of the recipes in this book at a moment's notice. They are all very minimal and quick to whip up (not including the occasional soaking time required).

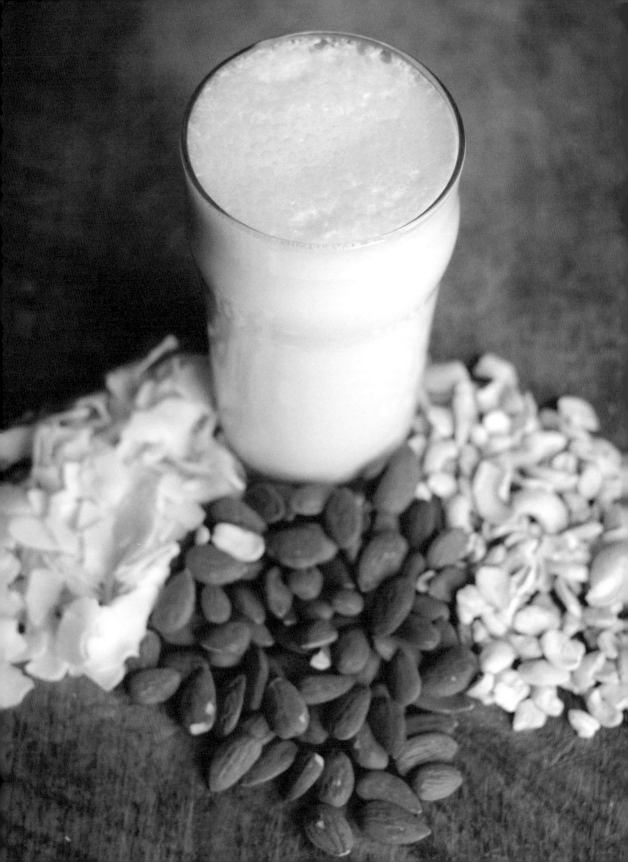

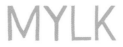

MYLK

Yield: 1 quart

Save your hard-earned dough, bypass the added sweeteners and sketchy preservatives, and make your own mylk! Spelled with a "y" as a reminder that it's nondairy.

PLAIN
¾ cup soaked nuts or seeds of choice
3 cups filtered water

NOURISHING
¾ cup soaked nuts or seeds of choice
3 cups Nourishing tea (p 3)

TIP: Feel free to experiment with other teas for varying flavor and health benefits.

VANILLA
Plain Mylk
1 tbsp vanilla extract
1–2 tbsp Date Paste (p 25) or liquid
    sweetener of choice (optional)
dash cinnamon (optional)

CHOCOLATE
Plain Mylk
3 tbsp raw cacao powder
1 tsp vanilla extract
1–2 tbsp Date Paste (p 25) or liquid
    sweetener of choice (optional)
dash of cinnamon (optional)

Combine soaked nuts or seeds of choice and water in a blender and blend for 30–60 seconds, until smooth. Pour mylk through a nut milk bag and gently squeeze as much liquid as you can into a bowl, jar, or pitcher. You can compost the pulp or save it for raw cookies, crackers, breads, or other fun creations! If you're not going to use it right away, you can freeze it for later.

For the flavored variations, once the base is made and strained, put it back into the blender with the remaining ingredients for the vanilla or chocolate mylk and blend for 15–30 seconds, or until thoroughly combined.

I keep plain mylk on hand to have a blank slate to start with when making various smoothies, hot drinks, etc. Lasts refrigerated for about 3 days.

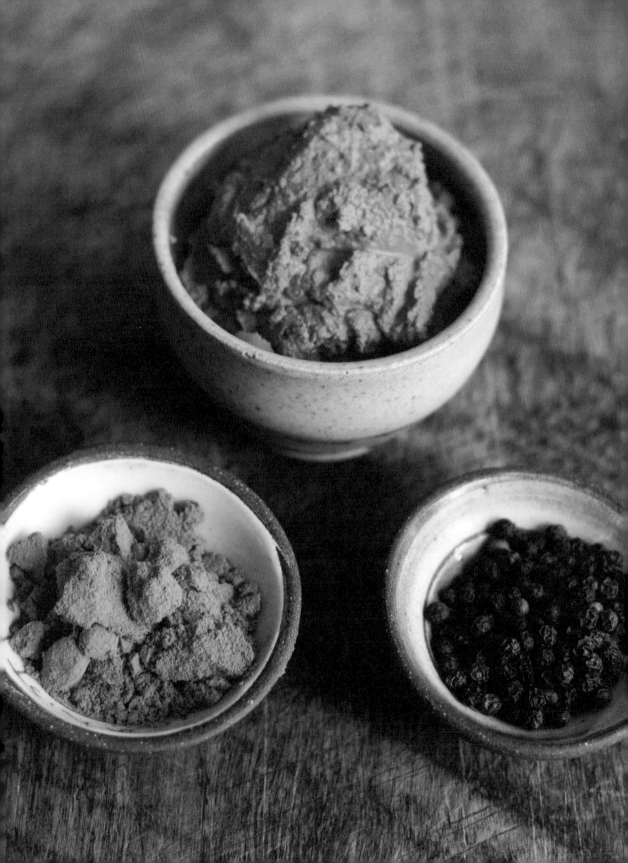

TURMERIC PASTE

Yield: 1 cup

The main base for the deliciously warming and wildly anti-inflammatory Golden Mylk (p 59) and Golden Goddess smoothie (p 135), turmeric paste is a wonderfully simple staple ingredient to have on hand.

To amplify the nutritional benefits of turmeric, we combine it with black pepper, as the piperine combines with the curcumin in turmeric to greatly amplify the benefits and make the curcumin tremendously more bioavailable (by 2,000 percent) for the human body to assimilate. Adding supplements and superfoods to your daily regimen is wonderful, but a waste if our bodies are not able to properly absorb them!

Don't worry, the pepper is such a minimal component in regards to the final taste of your drinks that you should barely notice it.

½ cup turmeric powder
1 cup filtered water
1 tsp ground black pepper

Put all ingredients into a small saucepan and cook over low heat, stirring until it has reached a paste-like consistency, approximately 3–5 minutes.

Let the mixture cool, then refrigerate in a sealed container. It should last for several weeks refrigerated.

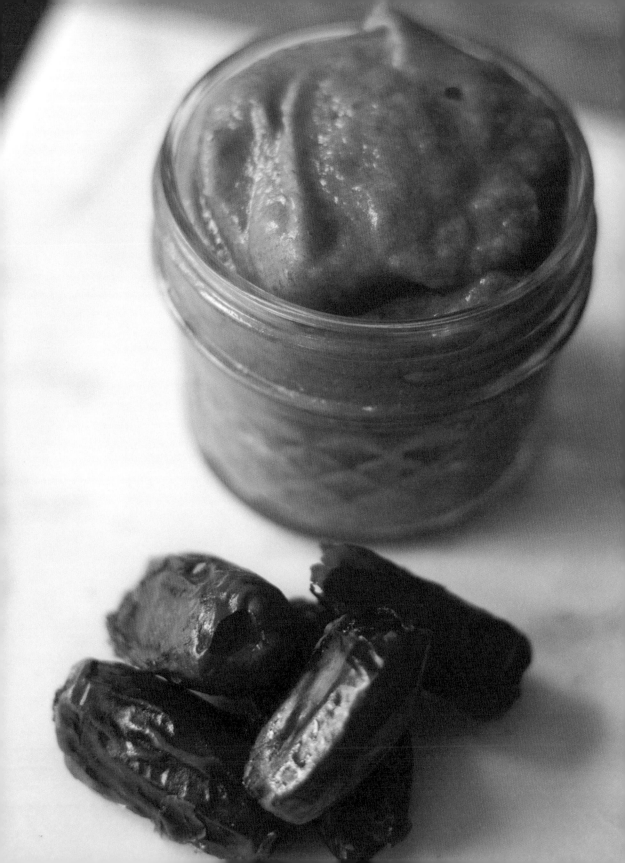

DATE PASTE

Yield: 3 cups

This is a great alternative sweetener to raw honey or maple syrup. While they still contain sugar, I find that dates offer my body a more well-balanced sugar experience that doesn't taste or feel as sweet. This is the sweetener I use most frequently. Date paste is raw (as opposed to maple syrup) and 100 percent vegan (unlike raw honey).

2 cups pitted deglet noor or medjool dates
Filtered water to cover

Even when labeled as pitted, you may still find some stragglers lingering, which your blender will highly disagree with (even a Vitamix or Blendtec). With that in mind, I recommend always cutting your dates in half to make sure there are no pits.

Cover the dates with filtered water and place them in the fridge, allowing them to soak for 8–12 hours or overnight. Blend the entire mixture into a smooth paste or leave as is and simply use the soaked dates anytime you'd use date paste (same amount). Date paste can be refrigerated in a sealed container for several weeks.

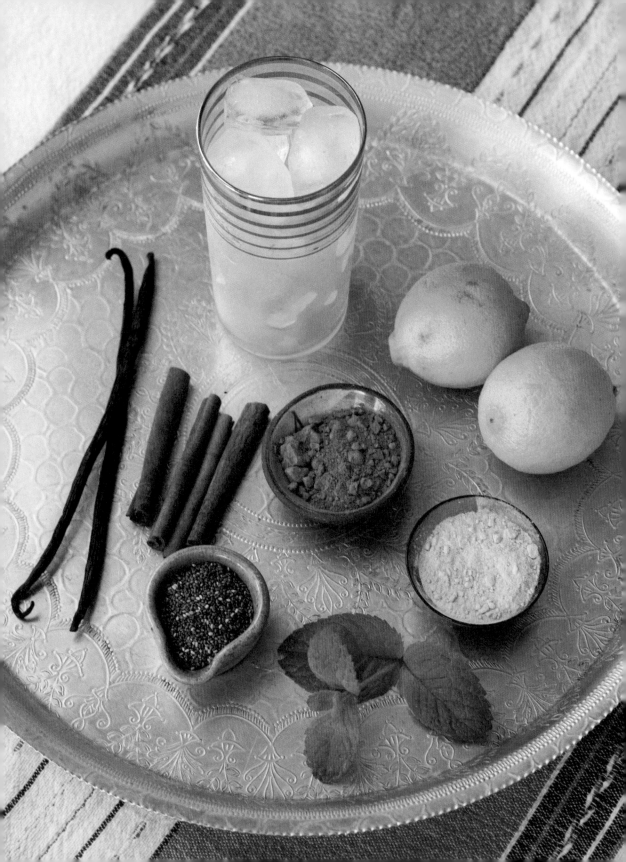

COOLING LIBATIONS

This chapter is designed for drinks that are less filling than smoothies and contain fiber and more concentrated protein than juice. These are perfect for cooling down in warmer weather or as light refreshments that deliver a powerful punch.

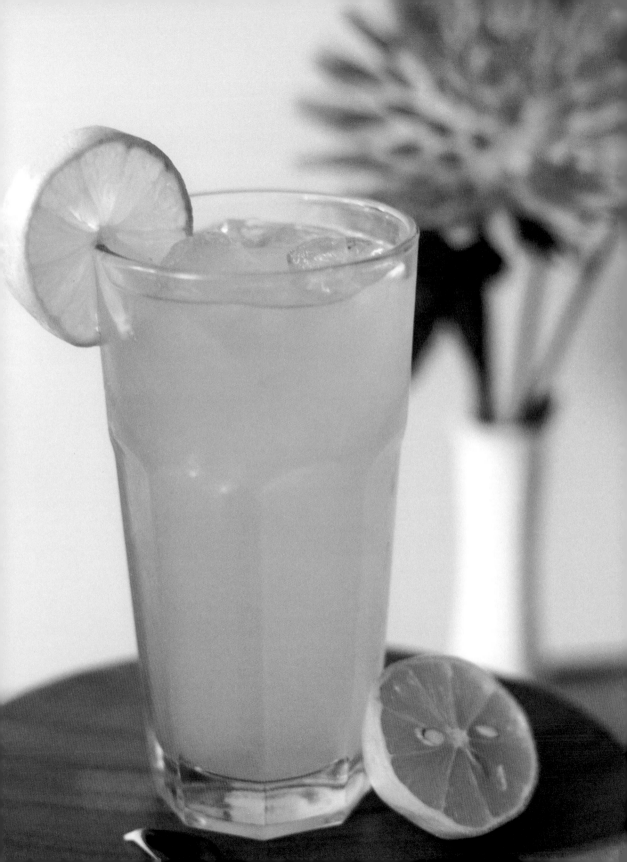

MAPLE LEMONADE

Yield: 2 cups

A popular summertime refreshment made simple and healthy with maple syrup as the sweetener. The earthy notes of the maple combine with the bright citrus in a beautiful balance.

The addition of cayenne quickly transforms this drink into the extra-cleansing backbone of the Master Cleanse, a liquid detox consisting only of this maple cayenne lemonade and a morning flush of salt water. Maple syrup is critical to this trendy cleanse, as it provides crucial vitamins and minerals that your body needs during such a restrictive time.

2½ tbsp pure maple syrup
2½ tbsp lemon juice (fresh-squeezed or concentrate)
1⅔ cups filtered or spring water

Make it a "master cleanser" by whisking in:
⅛ tsp cayenne pepper

Add all ingredients to a pitcher and stir until combined. Serve chilled, over ice if desired, and enjoy!

VARIATION: Feel free to use a favorite iced tea instead of filtered or spring water! Lemongrass is delicious and cooling!

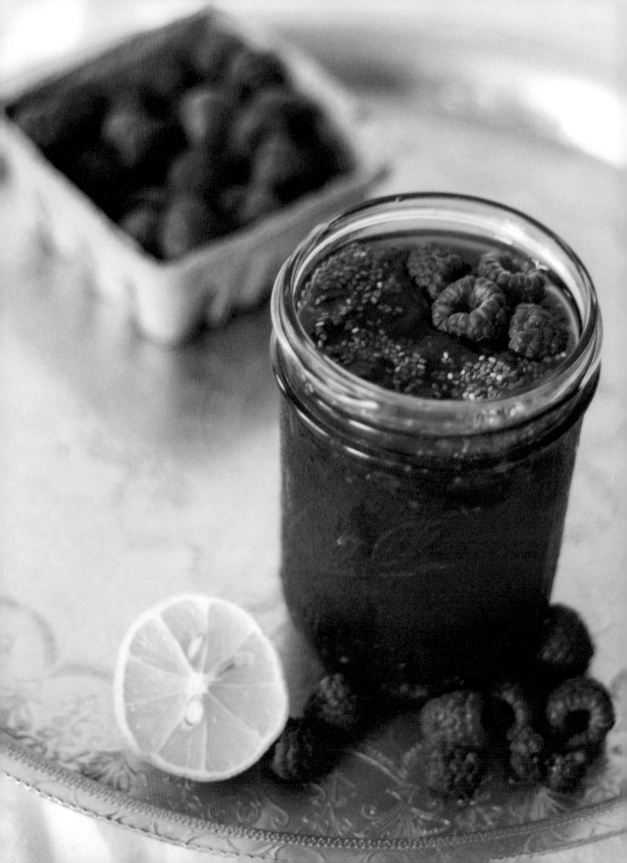

RASPBERRY CHIA LEMONADE

Yield: 2 cups

You may have seen some brands of kombucha that contain chia seeds on the shelves of your local health food store. Adding chia seeds to your water, fermented drink, juice, smoothie, etc. is a delicious and fun way to integrate these super seeds into your diet. Unlike adding seeds to a smoothie and blending, this recipe keeps the chia seeds intact, providing a playful texture reminiscent of bubble tea.

I use frozen raspberries in this recipe for a sweet, tart flavor pop!

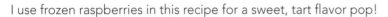

1¾ cups Maple Lemonade (p 29)
1 tbsp chia seeds
¼ cup frozen raspberries

Whisk together the Maple Lemonade and chia seeds in a pitcher. Serve over frozen raspberries and enjoy!

VARIATION: Feel free to try other frozen berries!

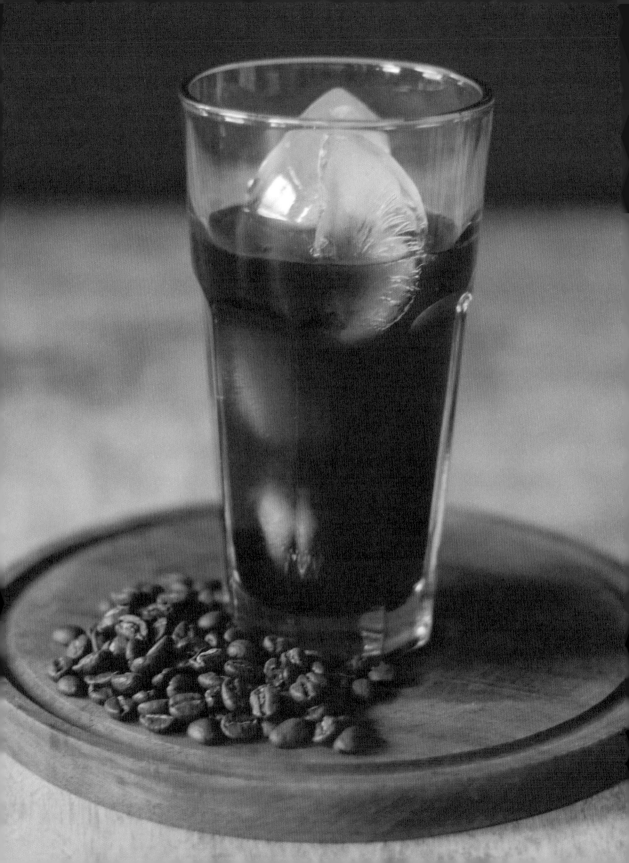

COLD BREW COFFEE

Smoother and 67 percent less acidic than your average cup o' Joe, you may never go back. You can even heat it up and drink it hot.

⅛ pound coffee beans, coarsely ground
4 cups filtered water

To make Cold Brew Concentrate, add coffee grounds and water to a glass jar and stir. Let steep at room temperature for 12 hours. Strain the coffee twice through a nut milk bag, fine-mesh sieve, or coffee filter. Dilute by combining equal parts filtered water and concentrate, then serve.* If desired, add mylk and sweetener to taste.

You can refrigerate the concentrate in a sealed container for up to 2 weeks. *Do not dilute until serving, as it will not last as long.

There are many at-home cold brew coffee systems you can use to cut down on the prep work and time, primarily the straining. See Equipment list (p 226) for more information.

> **TIP:** Generally speaking, cold brew coffee is brewed with cold or room temperature water. If you use hot water, it will speed up the brewing process and change the flavor profile. This may be handy when starting the cold brew late at night and it needs to be ready early in the morning (in less than 12 hours), but it will result in different flavor, strength, and acidity level.

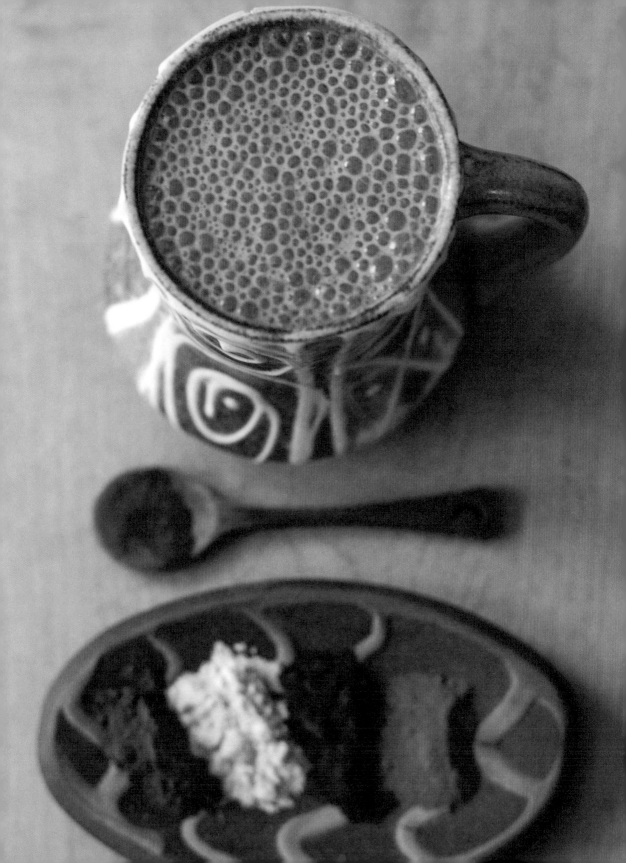

SUPER-HEROINE ICED COFFEE

Yield: 2 cups

I've named this the Super-Heroine for a few reasons: it is a cold, caffeinated twist on the Superhero Hot Chocolate (p 73); you will very quickly feel like a superhero after drinking it; and it is insanely addictive. The mixture of the coffee with the grounding adaptogenic herbs will recharge you and give you the strength to get through any day. You're welcome!

1 cup Cold Brew Coffee (p 33)
⅓ cup Mylk of choice (p 21)
3 tbsp raw cacao powder
1 tsp vanilla extract
1 tsp maca powder
¼ tsp shilajit extract
¼ tsp ashwagandha extract
¼ tsp holy basil extract
2 tbsp pure maple syrup
dash of cinnamon
several pieces of ice

Put all ingredients into a blender and blend until smooth. Enjoy the delicious jolt!

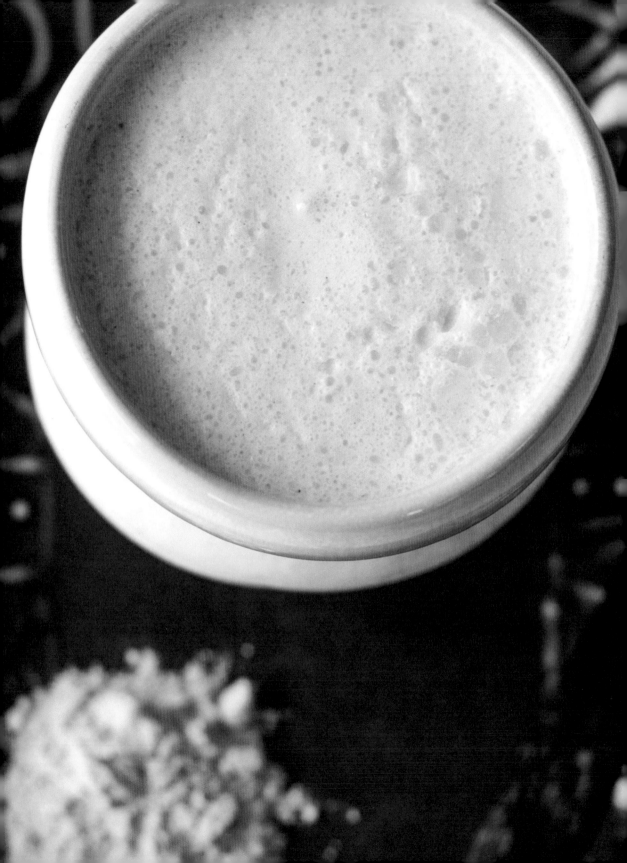

VANILLA MACA LOVE

Yield: 2 cups

I tell anyone who inquires about this drink at my café that it is like drinking a cloud (a crazy delicious cloud). While none of us will ever truly know what that is like, it doesn't take much imagination when drinking this to feel like this may be as close as you'll ever get to that sensation.

1½ cups mylk of choice
2 tsp vanilla extract
1 tsp maca powder
2 tbsp Date Paste (p 25)
dash of cinnamon
several pieces of ice

Put all ingredients into a blender and blend until the ice is broken down. Sip up, and be careful not to float away!

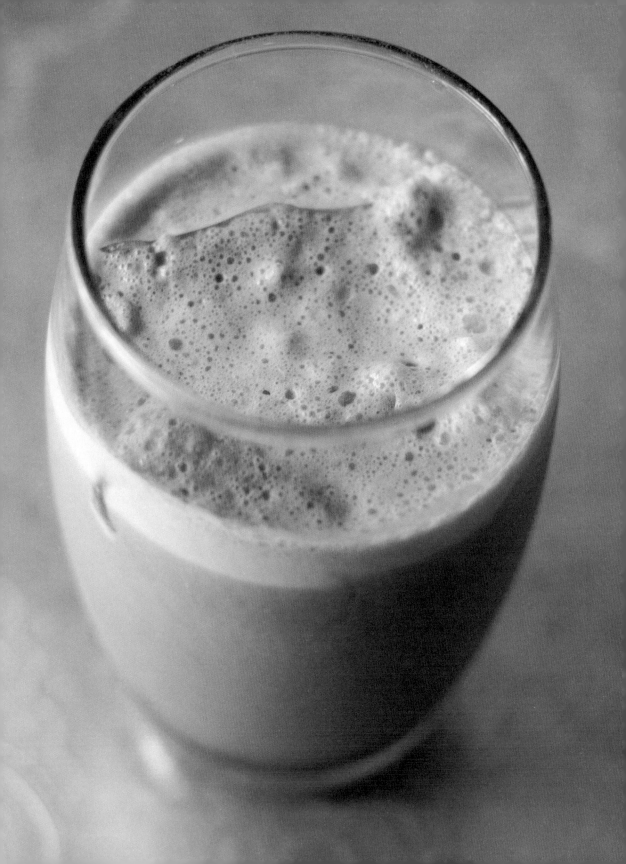

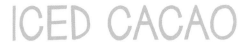

ICED CACAO

Yield: 2 cups

This is a simple superfood twist on classic chocolate mylk. Lucuma is a fruit that originates in Peru. In the dry, powdered form that we use, it adds a natural sweetness and an earthy, malty flavor that rounds out this cold drink.

1½ cups mylk of choice
2 tbsp raw cacao powder
1 tsp vanilla extract
2 tbsp Date Paste (p 25)
2 tsp lucuma powder
dash of cinnamon
several pieces of ice

Put all ingredients into a blender and blend until the ice is broken down. Enjoy!

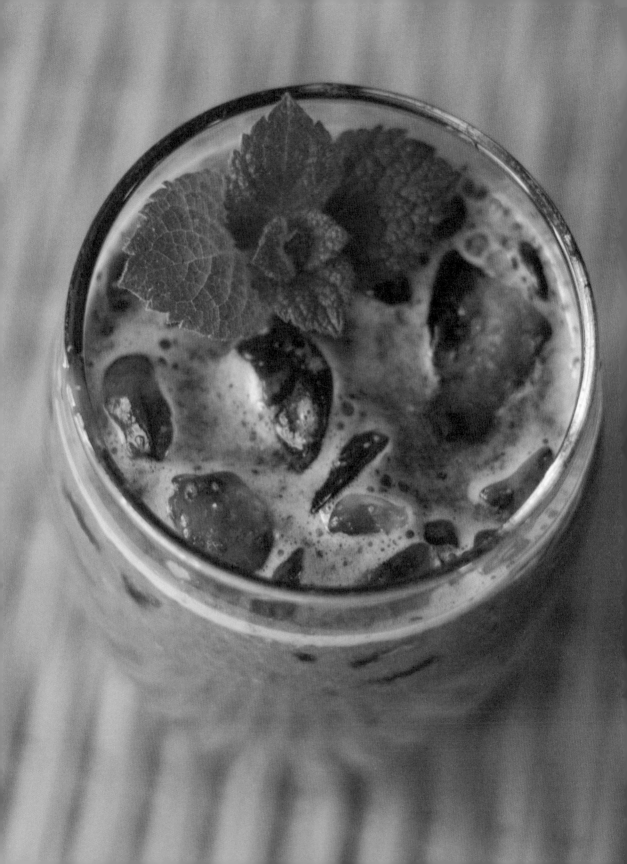

PEPPERMINT CHOCO-CHIA COOLER

Yield: 2 cups

I created this drink at the beginning of a shift at my Superfresh! Café. It was hot and humid outside, and I was feeling slightly lethargic. I needed a cooling boost of energy to get me through the day, and, as usual, I was craving chocolate. Luckily, our rotating iced herbal tea happened to be peppermint, which inspired this drink and made it so much easier to whip up.

Peppermint is both cooling and energizing; I use food-grade peppermint essential oil internally and externally when driving on long road trips to keep me awake and alert.

Chia seeds are an Aztec super seed. "Chia" is the Mayan word for "strength." Chia seeds increase stamina, boost energy, and are referred to as "Aztec running food."

¾ cup mylk of choice
¾ cup iced peppermint tea
2 tbsp raw cacao powder
1 tsp vanilla extract
1 tbsp chia seeds
2 tbsp Date Paste (p 25)
several pieces of ice

Put all ingredients into a blender and blend until the ice is broken down. Drink up, cool down, and feel your energy rise!

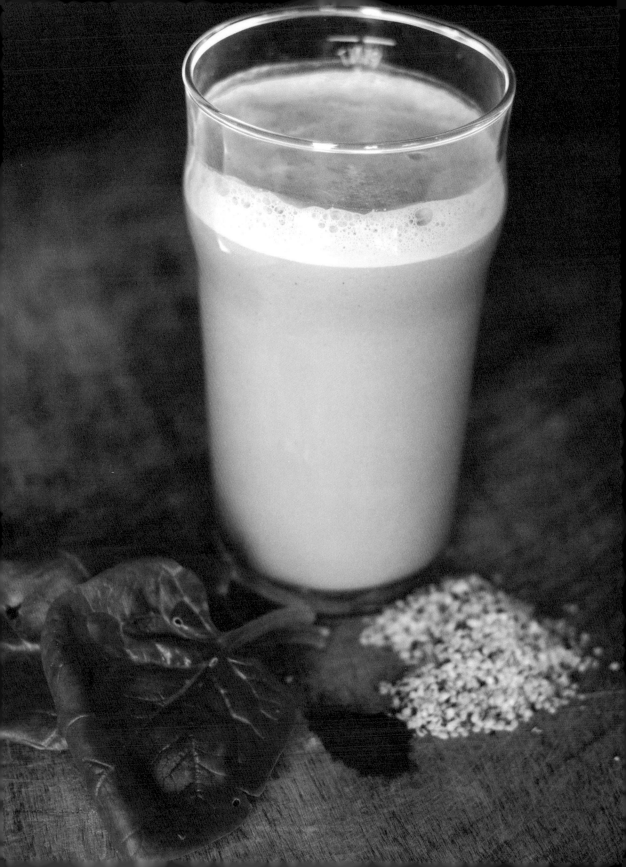

POPEYE POWER

I imagine this is what Popeye would gulp down if he had access to all the amazing superfoods we have at our fingertips today! More fibrous than a juice, less filling than a smoothie, this green mylk is filled with wonderful protein and green goodness that's sure to nourish your body and fuel you up for any endeavor.

1½ cups Nourishing Mylk (p 21) or mylk of choice
1 tbsp hemp seeds
handful of spinach
½ tsp spirulina
½ tsp vanilla extract
2 tbsp Date Paste (p 25)

Put all ingredients into a blender and blend until combined into a smooth mixture. Feel your body refuel and strengthen with each sip!

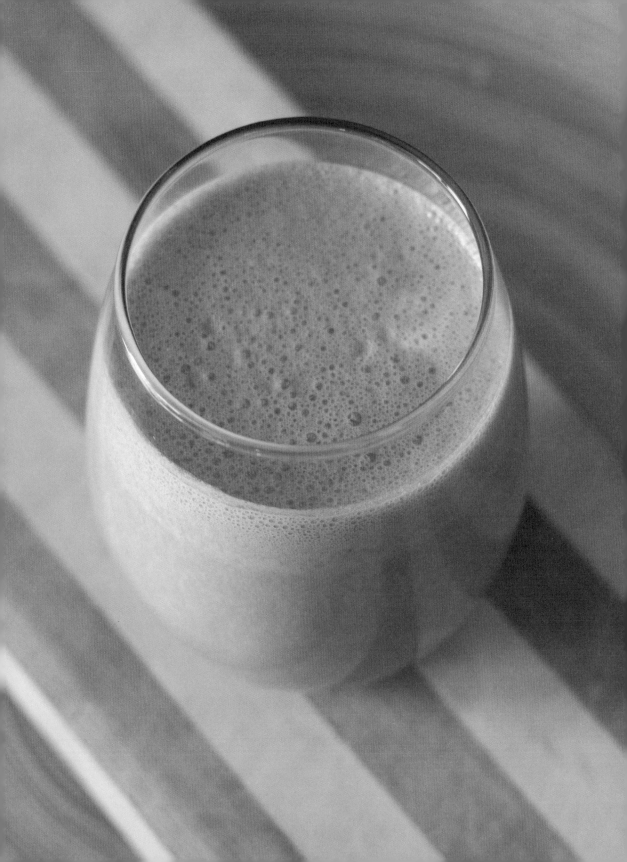

CHOCOLATE TEMPLE

Yield: 2 cups

This is the perfect superfood—chocolate mylk filled with some of my favorite herbal adaptogens and hemp seeds for an added protein boost. For those times when you don't want a hot drink, but still want to satisfy that chocolate craving.

1½ cups hemp mylk
3 tbsp raw cacao powder
1 tbsp hemp seeds
⅛ tsp shilajit extract powder
⅛ tsp holy basil extract powder
⅛ tsp ashwagandha extract powder
½ tsp vanilla extract
dash of cinnamon
2 tbsp Date Paste (p 25)
several pieces of ice

Put all ingredients into a blender and blend until creamy. Enjoy this luxurious blend!

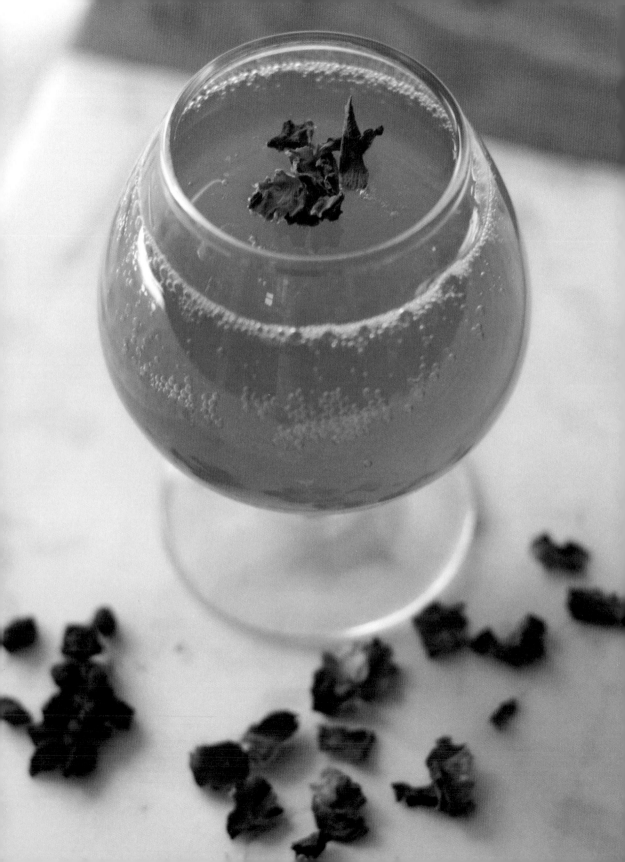

SCHISANDRA ROSE SPRITZER

Yield: 2 cups

A light and lovely sparkling drink that's perfect for sweetening any occasion.

1 cup filtered water
2 tsp schisandra berries
1 tbsp rose petals
2 tbsp raw honey
sparkling water to fill

In a medium saucepan bring the filtered water to a boil. Decrease heat to a simmer and add schisandra berries and rose petals. Cook down to a deep pink syrup, approximately 10 minutes. Remove the pan from the heat, then add the honey and stir well.

Allow to cool. Pour into two fancy flutes or wine glasses, top with sparkling water, and toast to love!

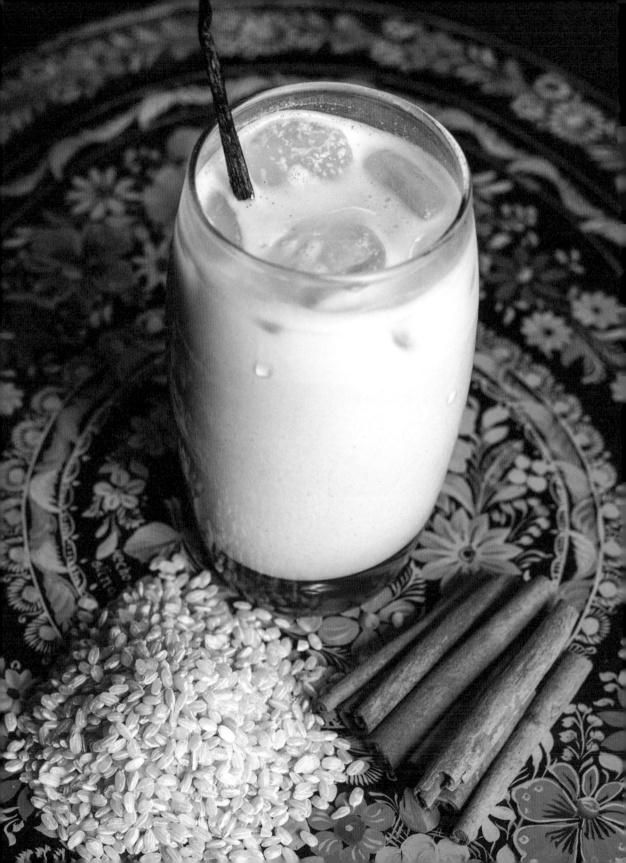

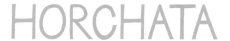

HORCHATA

Yield: 2 cups

This Mexican *agua fresca* reminds me of cooling down on hot, humid summer days. It is light, creamy, smooth, and delicious!

½ cup uncooked, dry brown rice
4 cups filtered water
4 tbsp Date Paste (p 25) or liquid sweetener of choice
1 tsp cinnamon
1 tsp vanilla extract

Put the rice and 2 cups of the water into a blender and blend until the rice begins to break down, approximately 1 minute. Pour the mixture into a bowl or jar, add the remaining 2 cups of water, and allow to sit at room temperature for 3 hours or overnight.

Pour the mixture into the blender and blend until smooth. Strain the rice water through a nut milk bag or cheesecloth into a pitcher. Discard the rice.

Add the rice water to the blender with the date paste, cinnamon, and vanilla. Blend. Chill and stir. Serve over ice and enjoy!

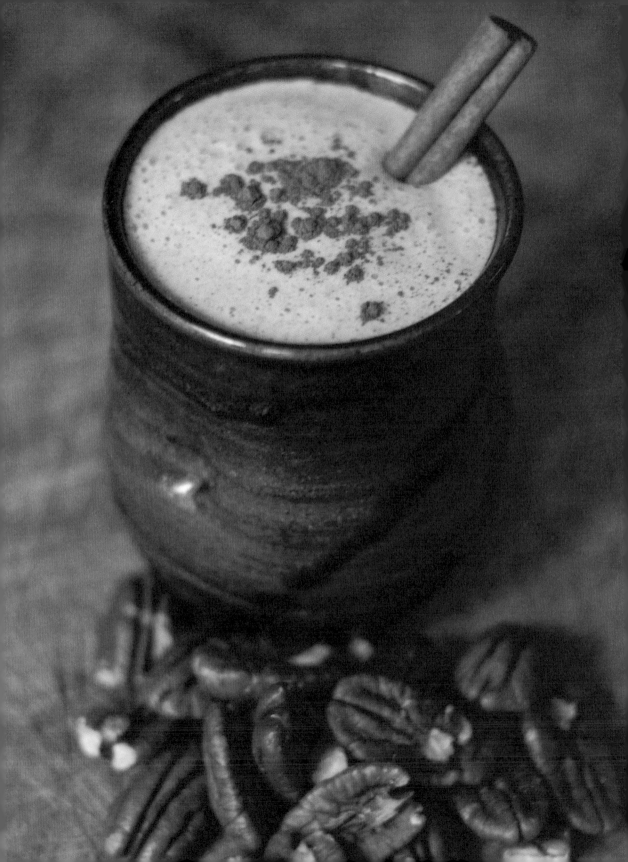

'NOG

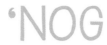

Yield: 2 cups

One of the hardest things about living with dietary restrictions can be the social element, especially around the holidays. With this recipe you'll no longer be left out of enjoying the 'nog experience at the holiday party—you may even be the showstopper and convert many questioning bystanders. This is truly vegan Christmas heaven (or Chanukah, winter solstice, etc.).

1⅓ cups mylk of choice
⅓ cup pecans
1 tsp cinnamon
¼ tsp nutmeg
1 tsp vanilla extract
2 tbsp Date Paste (p 25)
several pieces of ice

Blend all ingredients together and enjoy the yuletide spirit!

TIP: Add a shot of brandy, rum, or bourbon if you desire. For added healing benefits, add 1-2 ounces of chaga concentrate, or make mylk with Medicinal Mushroom Tea (p 5).

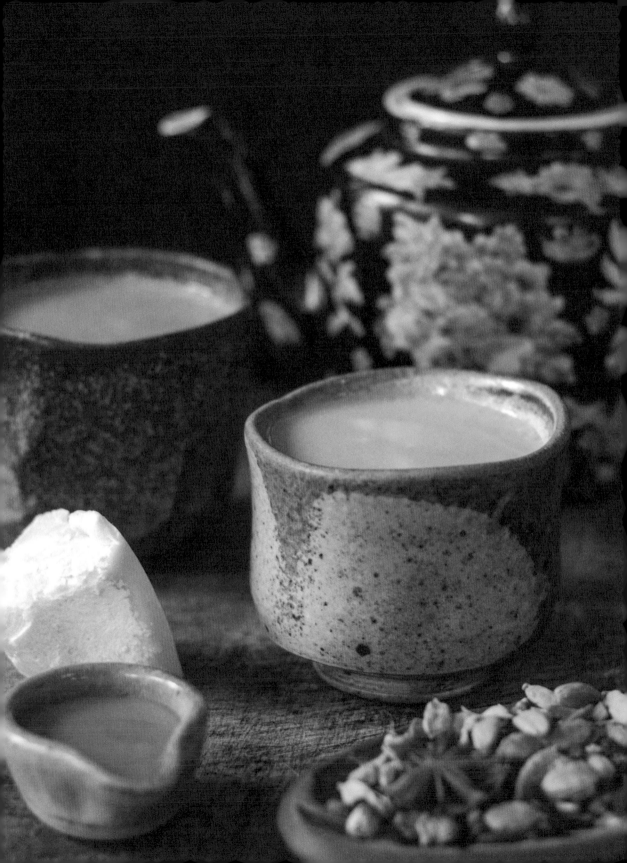

HOT ELIXIRS

While concocting any of the beverages in this book (and beyond) provides a beautifully sacred ritualistic experience, I find that the Hot Elixirs definitely stand out more so in this regard. Perhaps that is because they are also warming, and therefore extra heart nourishing in that warmth.

There are recipes in this chapter for zapping illness, reducing inflammation, preventative care, relaxing and calming your body and mind, grounding your energy, stimulating your spirit, and more.

I have found that when I am not drinking coffee the thing I miss the most is my morning ritual of boiling water, grinding beans, and making the pour rather than the caffeine jolt. Converting from coffee to superfood elixirs allows you to keep that physical practice with a more healing outcome.

TIP: Substitute tea for hot water in any of these recipes. The chocolate and chai drinks are also insanely delicious with coffee as the hot liquid! I go a little health crazy and brew my pour-over coffee with a healing tea (usually Nourishing or Medicinal Mushroom) and then add superfoods on top of that! Have FUN!

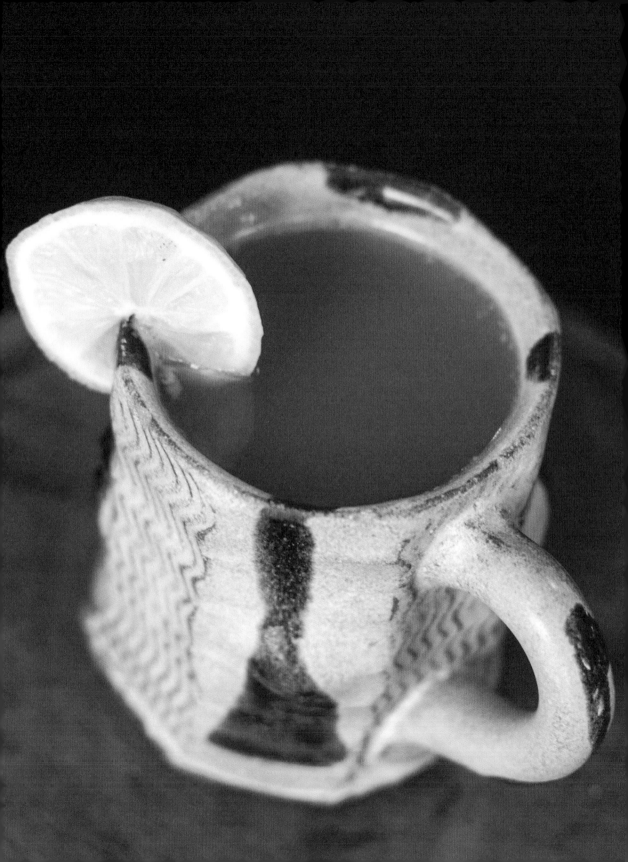

SORE THROAT SOOTHER

Yield: 2 cups

If you are sick, and especially if you have a sore throat, this recipe is a surefire way to boost your body back to wellness and soothe your pain. Extremely strong, this will both soothe and warm your entire being almost immediately.

I normally suggest using another sweetener of choice or say that the sweetener is optional, however the healing benefits of raw honey in this specific beverage (especially because of what it is geared toward) is unmatched with other options. If you are hardcore vegan, I recommend simply leaving the honey out instead of using a different sweetener, as the benefits of this potent brew will still be great. If you really need to add sweetener to offset the potency, maple syrup would be my next best recommendation. Note: The honey in this recipe is not included for flavor, but rather for its medicinal qualities.

⅓ cup apple cider vinegar
⅓ cup lemon juice
2 inches fresh ginger root, sliced
1½ cups filtered water
2 tbsp raw honey
⅛ tsp cayenne pepper (optional)

Put the vinegar, lemon juice, ginger root, and water into a small saucepan and cook over low heat for about 10 minutes. This is not something you want to leave too long, as the vinegar will lose its potency and medicinal benefits when cooked at length. Once it reaches the desired temperature, remove from heat, strain into a mug, add the honey and cayenne, if desired, and slowly sip in the healing.

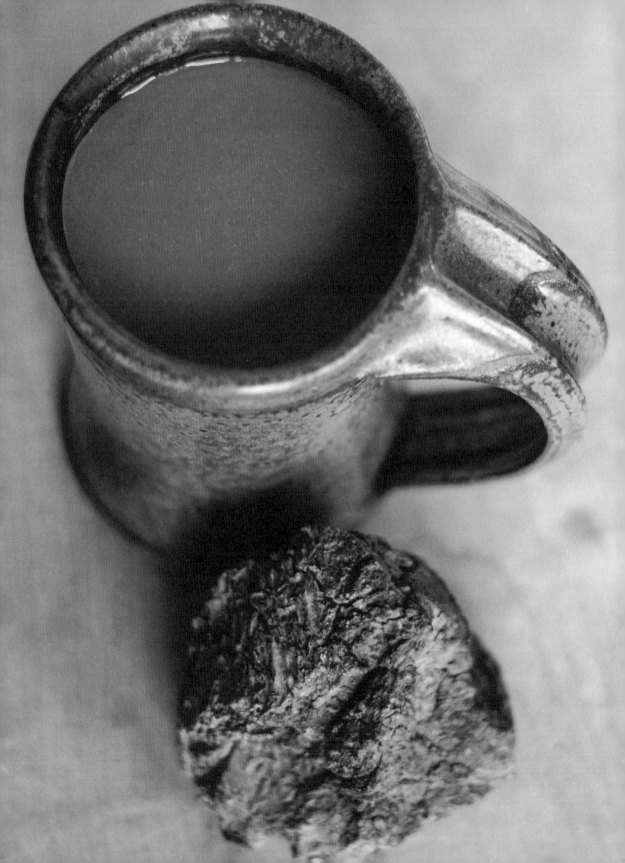

CHICORY CHAGA CAFÉ

If you're looking for a coffee alternative, this is a wonderful medicinal blend that provides a dark, earthy, grounding, bitter brew that makes a great option. The medicinal benefits include improving digestion, boosting immunity, and cleansing the liver.

1 tbsp chaga powder
3½ cups water
1 tbsp roasted chicory root
1 tbsp roasted dandelion root
1 cinnamon stick
½ cup coconut mylk (optional)
2 tbsp raw honey or liquid sweetener of choice (optional)

Add chaga and water to a medium saucepan and bring to a boil. Reduce heat to low-medium and brew for 20–30 minutes. Add chicory, dandelion, and cinnamon and steep for another 5 minutes.

Strain liquid into desired mug, then add mylk and sweetener.

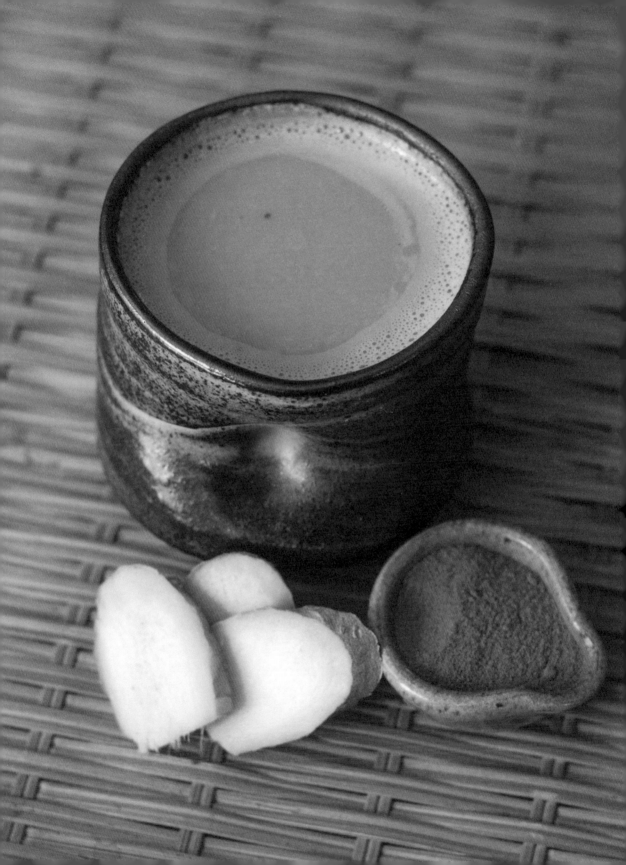

GOLDEN MYLK

Yield: 2 cups

This Ayurvedic classic has recently received much attention and has been making its way into the Western world by being featured in health food cafés, prepackaged beverages, and numerous blogs. The backbone of this drink is the popular Indian spice of turmeric, which is one of the most medicinal spices known for its anti-inflammatory powers (see p 249 for more details).

Ginger and vanilla extract are added to this recipe to round out the flavor profile and amplify the healing benefits.

½ cup coconut mylk
1½ tsp Turmeric Paste (p 23)
1 tsp vanilla extract
1 tsp ginger juice
2 tbsp raw honey or liquid sweetener of choice (optional)
1½ cups hot water

Blend the coconut mylk, turmeric paste, vanilla extract, ginger juice, and honey together. Pour the concentrate into your favorite mug, fill with hot water, and enjoy.

TIP: While in many recipes I say to use your choice of mylk, I've found that this Golden Mylk recipe really is best with the creamy fattiness of coconut mylk.

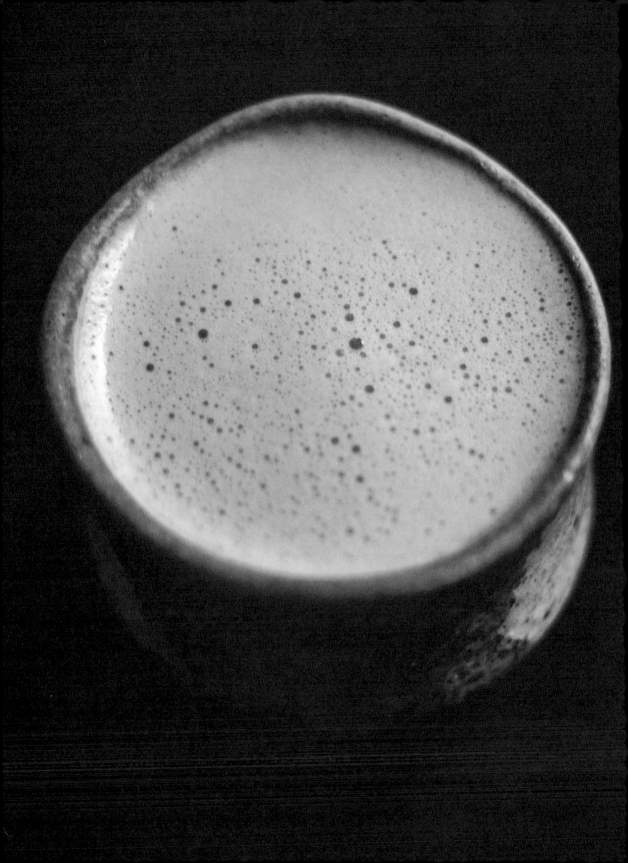

MATCHA LATTÉ

Yield: 2 cups

This warming, earthy, creamy green drink delivers a delicious caffeinated kick filled with powerful antioxidants sure to boost your overall health and carry you through your day with clean energy.

½ cup Mylk (p 21)
1 tsp matcha green tea powder
1 tsp vanilla extract
2 tbsp raw honey or liquid sweetener of choice (optional)
1½ cups hot water

Blend together the mylk, matcha green tea powder, vanilla extract, and honey. Pour the concentrate into your favorite mug, fill with hot water, and enjoy!

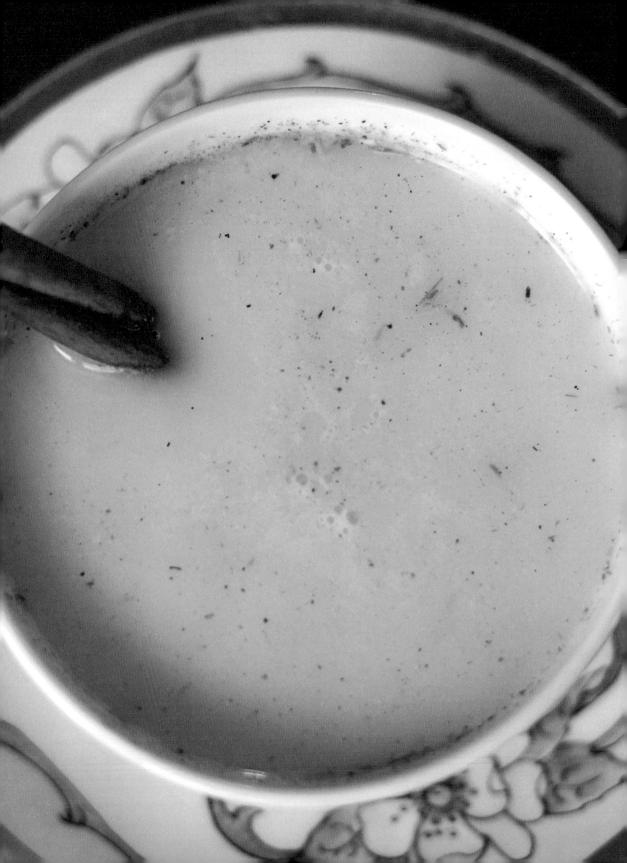

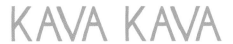

KAVA KAVA

Yield: 2 cups

Kava is a root originating from Polynesia (often used in ceremonies there) with very potent nervine qualities that will relax your body almost immediately to varying degrees based on variety and quantity consumed.

Just as a heads-up, kava is so powerful that with as little as one sip you'll likely feel your tongue go numb. This is normal. Enjoy!

½ cup Mylk (p 21)
1 tsp kava kava powder
1½ cups hot water
dash of cinnamon

Blend together the mylk and kava kava powder. Pour the concentrate into your favorite mug, fill with hot water, garnish with cinnamon, and enjoy!

TIP: This is also delicious iced and served with a slice of pineapple garnish. Add 1-2 ounces of chaga concentrate or make mylk with Medicinal Mushroom Tea (p 5) for an added depth of healing benefits.

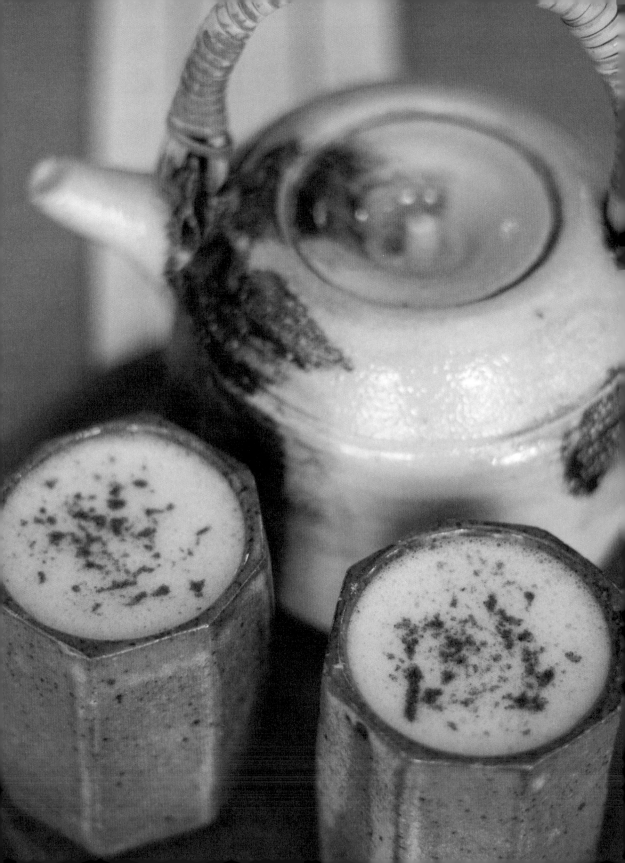

CHAMOMILE CARDAMOM KAVA

Yield: 2 cups

This deliciously rounded, earthy brew combines the calming benefits of chamomile and kava with the soulful sensations of cardamom, also extremely healing in its own right. I greatly enjoy this elixir at the end of a long day to help relax me into sweet slumber in conjunction with an Epsom salt bath filled with my favorite essential oils with candles glowing, or as a soothing reset button during stressful, anxiety-filled times.

1½ cups hot chamomile tea
½ cup Mylk (p 21)
½ tsp cardamom powder
½ tsp kava kava powder
1 tsp vanilla extract
2 tbsp raw honey or liquid sweetener of choice (optional)

Brew the chamomile tea. Blend together the mylk, cardamom powder, kava kava powder, vanilla extra, and honey. Pour the concentrate into your favorite mug, top off with the hot tea, and enjoy!

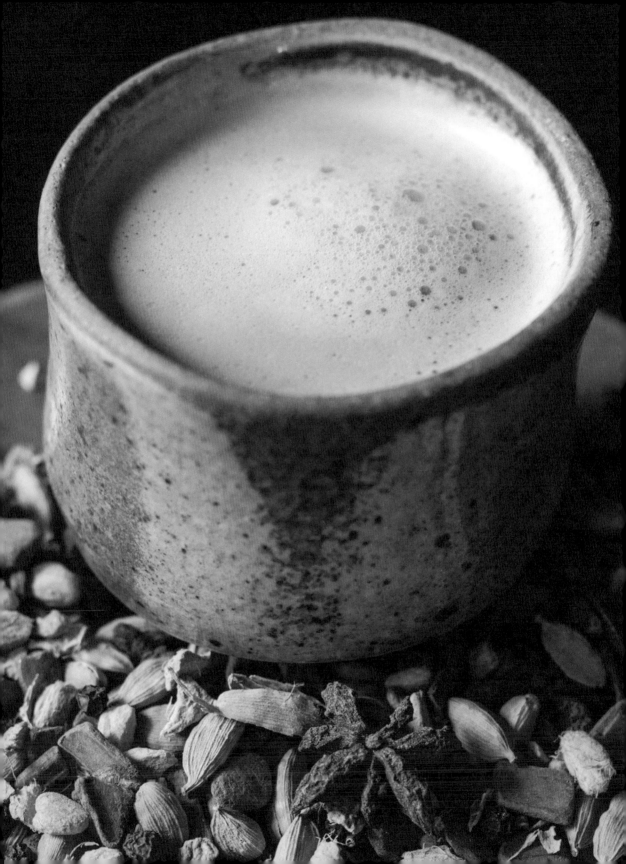

CHAGA CHAI

Yield: 2 cups

Chai is a cherished healing elixir that has been beloved in India for centuries. It is known to increase health and ease the mind. This recipe is recommended as caffeine-free and begins with a strong brew of chaga tea to amplify the healing benefits to a whole new level. Feel free to brew with the addition of black tea for an added caffeinated jolt.

CHAI CONCENTRATE:

½ tsp chaga powder
1-inch piece fresh ginger root
3–4 cardamom pods
3 whole cloves
¼ tsp whole black peppercorn
1 whole star anise
3½ cups filtered water

2 tsp black tea (optional)
½ cup mylk of choice (I prefer thicker mylks for this, such as coconut, cashew, or almond mylk)
1 tsp extra virgin coconut oil
2 tbsp raw honey or liquid sweetener of choice (optional)

Put the chaga powder, ginger, cardamom, cloves, peppercorn, star anise, and water in a medium saucepan and bring to a boil. Reduce heat to low-medium and brew for 20–30 minutes, longer if you'd like a stronger cup. If you'd like to add black tea for caffeine, add at the end and let steep for about 3 minutes.

Strain the liquid into a blender and add mylk, coconut oil, and sweetener. Blend on low for 5–10 seconds. Pour into your favorite mug and enjoy!

ICE IT: This drink is also extremely delicious iced (for this version I usually swap honey for maple syrup and leave out the coconut oil).

TIP: Brew a big pot of chai concentrate and store in a sealed jar in your fridge to use when desired. Chaga is a natural antibacterial, prolonging the life of this beverage.

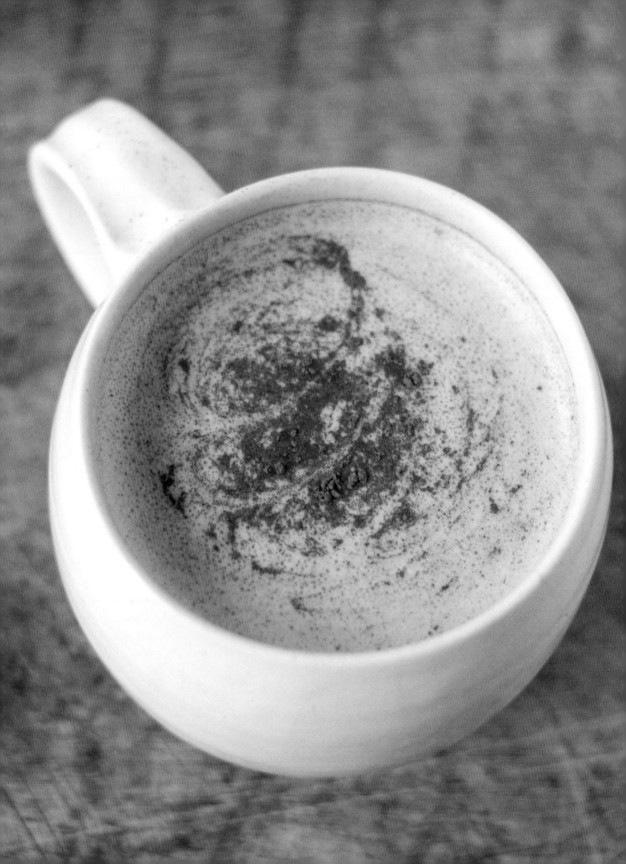

SHILAJIT LATTÉ

Yield: 2 cups

This elixir is gorgeously grounded with an earthy dose of Ayurvedic adaptogens perfectly blended to carry you through dreary winter months and stressful times.

The trifecta of Shilajit, holy basil, and ashwagandha is one of my staple superfood combos. I add it to so many of my drinks and always have a jar of it preblended and ready to go! Shilajit, nicknamed the "Destroyer of Weaknesses," is a mineral extract from the Himalayas; when taken in conjunction with other Ayurvedic herbs their benefits are said to be tenfold.

½ cup Mylk (p 21)
⅛ tsp shilajit extract powder
⅛ tsp holy basil extract powder
⅛ tsp ashwagandha extract powder
1 tsp vanilla extract
2 tbsp raw honey or liquid sweetener of choice (optional)
1½ cups hot water
dash of cinnamon

Blend together the mylk, shilajit, holy basil, ashwagandha, vanilla, and sweetener of choice. Pour the concentrate into your favorite mug, fill with hot water, garnish with cinnamon, and enjoy!

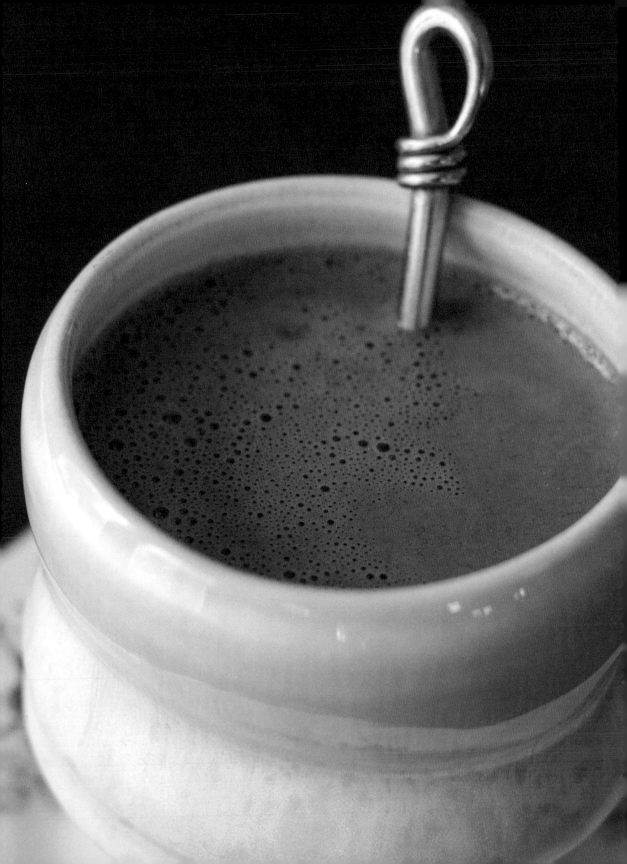

BASIC HOT CHOCOLATE

Yield: 2 cups

Everyone needs a classic hot chocolate recipe to replace that old sugar-filled mix in your cabinet. This recipe is insanely simple, while also being an amazing base for endless possibilities!

½ cup Mylk (p 21)
3 tbsp raw cacao powder or ceremonial cacao
2 tbsp pure maple syrup or liquid sweetener of choice (optional)
1 tsp vanilla extract (optional)
1½ cups hot water

PEPPERMINT:
½ tsp peppermint extract

SPICY:
⅛ tsp cayenne pepper
dash of cinnamon

Blend together the mylk, cacao, sweetener of choice, and vanilla. For the Peppermint or Spicy version, combine the additional ingredients into the mix. Pour the concentrate into your favorite mug, fill with hot water, and enjoy!

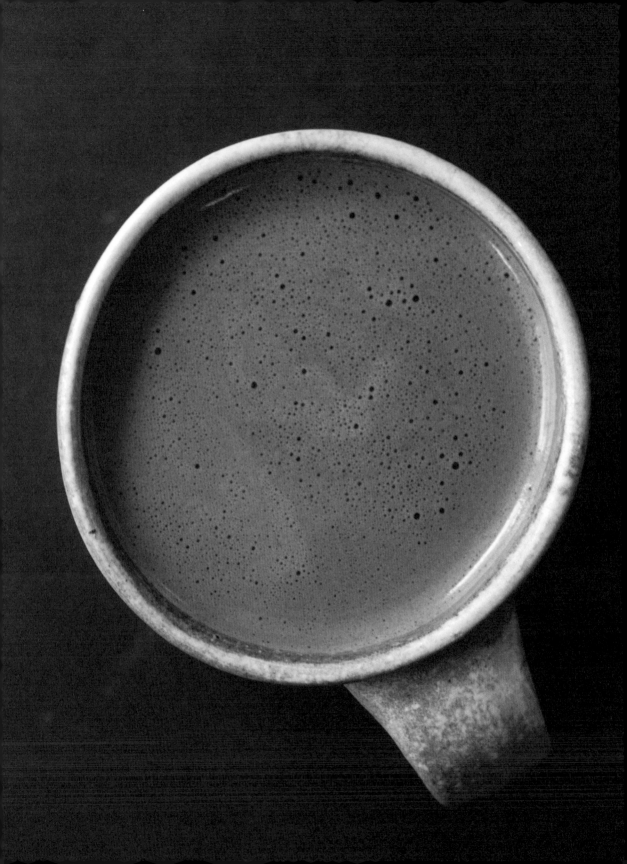

SUPERHERO HOT CHOCOLATE

Yield: 2 cups

This is my absolute favorite superfood chocolate elixir that always makes life just a little bit—or a lot—better.

½ cup Mylk (p 21)
3 tbsp raw cacao powder
1½ tsp lucuma powder
1½ tsp maca powder
⅛ tsp shilajit extract powder
1 tsp vanilla extract
1½ tbsp raw honey or liquid sweetener of choice (optional)
dash of cinnamon
1½ cups hot water

Combine the mylk, cacao, lucuma, maca, shilajit, vanilla, sweetener of choice, and cinnamon. Pour the concentrate into your favorite mug, fill with hot water, and enjoy!

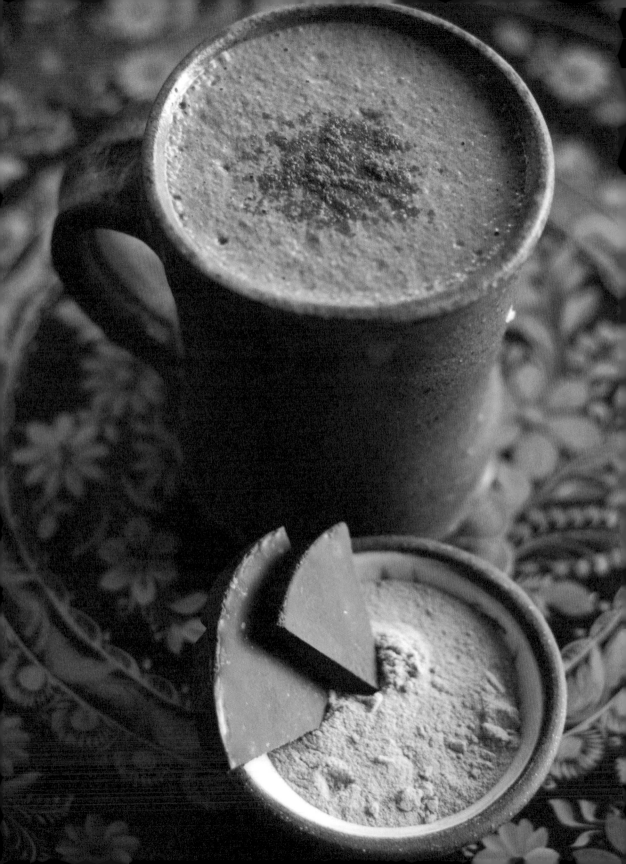

XOCOLATL

(pronounced sho-co-lot)

Yield: 2 cups

In Aztec culture, cacao was primarily consumed as the drink *xocolatl*, translated as "bitter water," by warriors and the elite. This Xocolatl recipe utilizes ceremonial cacao with the added heat of cayenne and the delicious, sweet, nutty notes of mesquite.

Ceremonial cacao is more bitter than its raw counterpart, which is sweeter and smoother. It is prepared with traditional Mayan techniques of fermenting and lightly roasting the beans.

½ cup Mylk (p 21)
3 tbsp ceremonial cacao block*,
    shaved or grated
1 tsp mesquite powder
1 tsp vanilla extract
⅛ tsp cayenne pepper
2 tbsp raw honey or liquid sweetener of
    choice (optional)

1½ cups hot water
dash of cinnamon
*Feel free to swap for raw cacao powder if you
    don't have ceremonial or simply prefer a
    smoother, less bitter taste.*

Combine the mylk, cacao, mesquite powder, vanilla, cayenne and honey. Pour the concentrate into your favorite mug, fill with hot water, add a dash of cinnamon, and enjoy!

TIP: Ceremonial cacao can also be prepared over the stove in a small saucepan, melting the cacao in with water on low heat and stirring occasionally. When made on the stovetop following traditional ceremonial preparations, this drink has an extremely thick, sludge-like consistency. See Sourcing (p 230) to find my recommended link with more information.

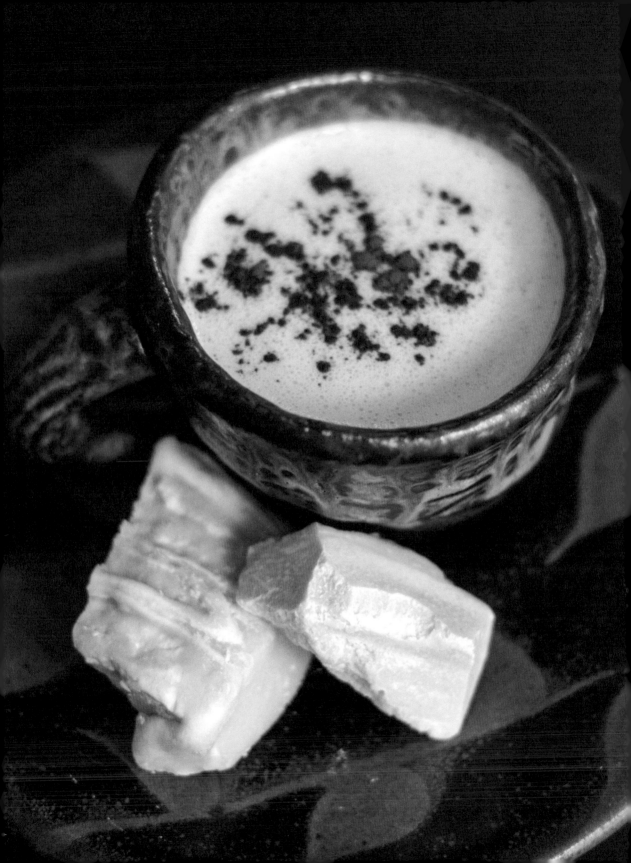

WHITE HOT CHOCOLATE

Yield: 2 cups

This White Hot Chocolate is frothy, silky, creamy, and ideal on those bitter cold, picture-perfect, winter wonderland snow globe days.

3 tbsp cacao butter
½ cup Mylk (p 21)
¼ cup raw cashews
1 tsp vanilla extract
1½ tbsp raw honey or liquid sweetener of choice (optional)
½ tsp peppermint extract (optional)
1½ cups hot water

Combine the cacao butter, mylk, cashews, and vanilla extract. If desired, add the honey and/or the peppermint extract. Pour the concentrate into your favorite mug, then fill with hot water. Sip by the fireplace for ultimate enjoyment.

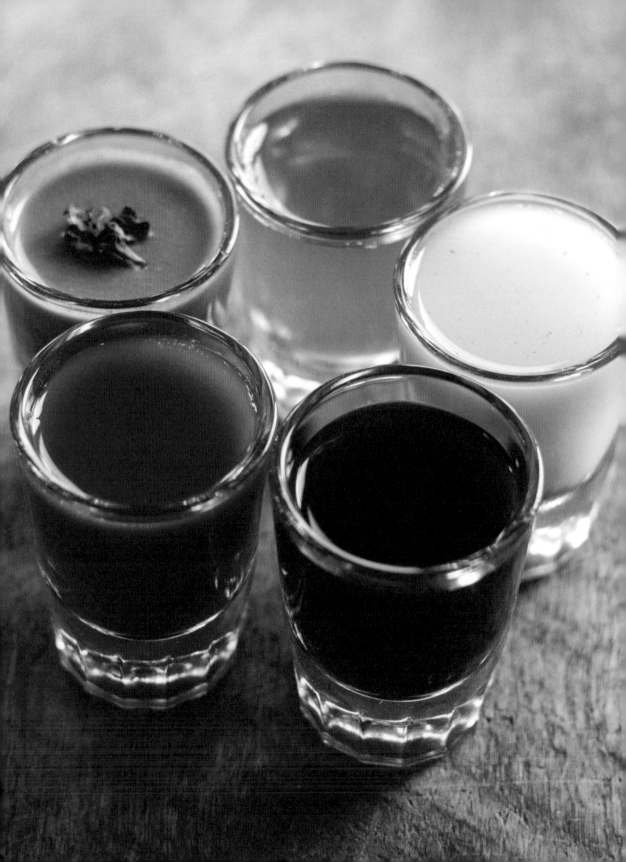

POWER-PACKED SHOTS

These tiny tonics pack a potent punch in as little as one to two ounces!

In this case, more is not always better. A little bit goes quite a long way, and overdoing it can have negative side effects depending on the recipe, dosage, and your physical needs. Think of homeopathy: less is more, and more can actually be harmful. For instance, drinking more than 8–12 ounces of wheatgrass a day (unless working with a health professional for a very specific and regulated reason) is simply overkill, and usually our bodies are unable to absorb that much at a time. Honestly, 1–2 ounces a day and you'll be flying higher than most!

Integrate these shots as guided into your health regime for daily preventative care, relief from sickness, or as a special pick-me-up.

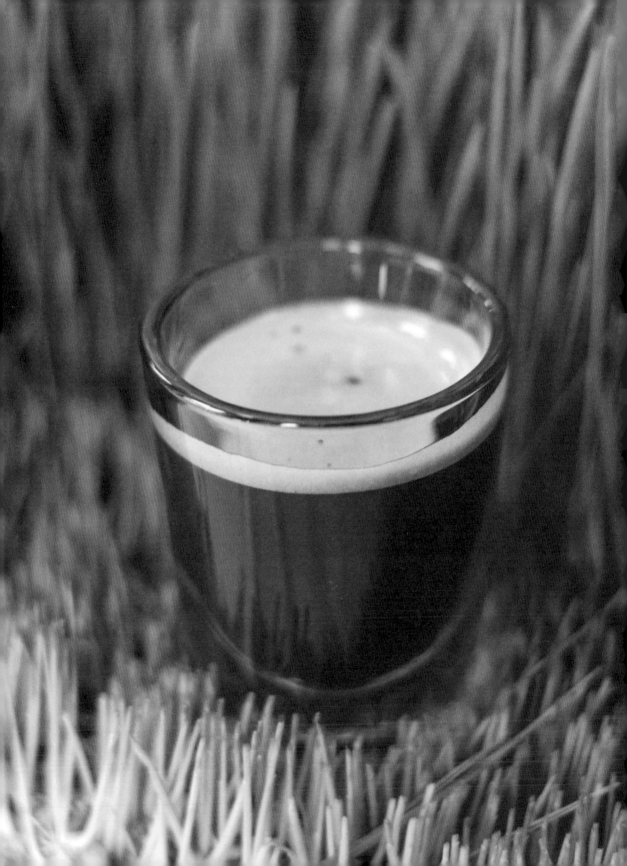

WHEATGRASS

Yield: 2 ounces

Wheatgrass is hands down the healthiest juice on the scene and is argued to be all you need to survive. It is made up of 70 percent chlorophyll, which is called the blood of the plant, as it has a molecular structure almost identical to the hemoglobin molecule of human blood. It is nutritionally complete, containing all known minerals, 17 amino acids, and is extremely rich in protein. This grass assimilates into the bloodstream within 20 minutes with very little energy.

Don't be deceived by the name; while wheatgrass is indeed the same plant that wheat berries come from, it does not contain gluten. Gluten is a protein found specifically in the wheat berry and other grains, such as rye, spelt, and barley.

¼ pound wheatgrass
orange wedge (optional)

Use a wheatgrass juicer to extract the juice from your wheatgrass. Shoot it down, and chase it with an orange wedge to help ease the punch.

> **TIP:** If you do not have a wheatgrass juicer, a masticating juicer can also handle wheatgrass; unfortunately, centrifugal juicers will not work. You can also use a manual wheatgrass juicer instead of the more expensive electric variety—see the Equipment chapter (p 226) for more information.
>
> You can also find raw, dehydrated wheatgrass powder at your local health food store or online.

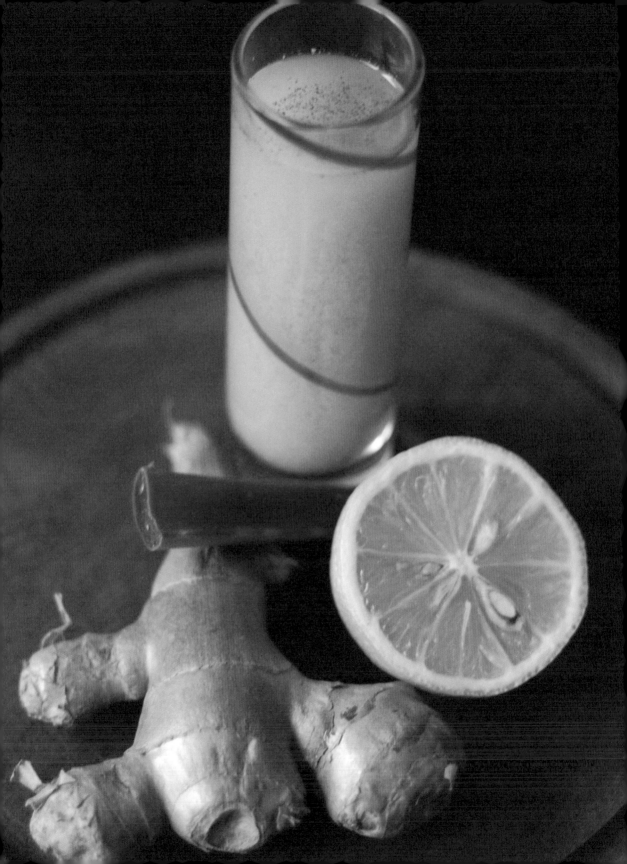

GINGER ALOE LEMON

Yield: 2 ounces

This immune-boosting shot can be used as a healthy skin tonic, a hangover helper, or a quick pick-me-up.

1 oz aloe juice
½ oz lemon juice (fresh or concentrate)
½ oz ginger juice
¼ tsp cayenne pepper (optional)

Add all ingredients to a measuring cup and whisk until combined. Pour into a shot glass and drink up!

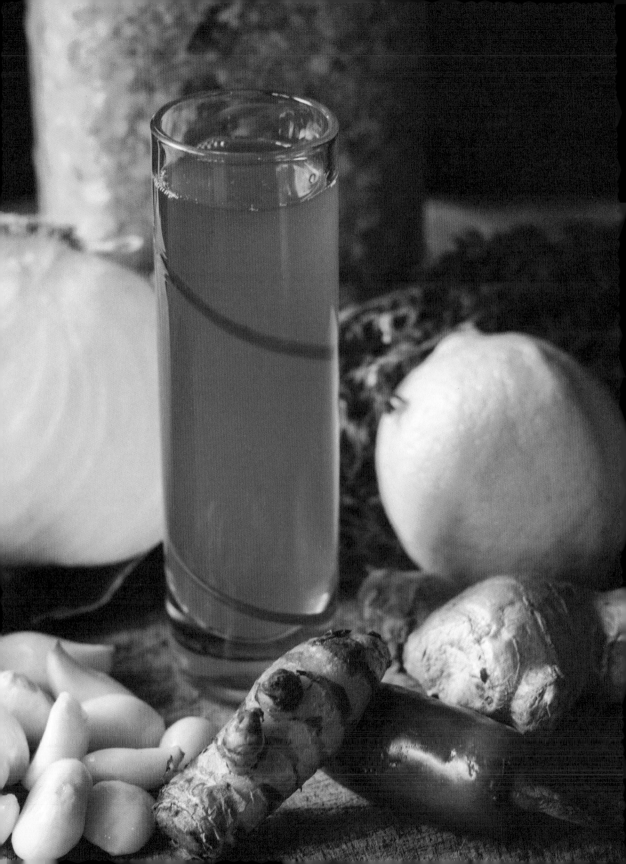

SUMMER GARDEN FIRE TONIC

Yield: approximately 1 quart

Fire cider is a key component to the herbal medicine cabinet. It is a vinegar infusion mixed with raw honey that is most used during the winter months / flu season for its potent immune-boosting properties. Making your own at home is very easy.

juice and zest from 1 lemon
½ cup fresh ginger root, grated or minced
½ cup horseradish root, grated
10 garlic cloves, minced
1 medium onion, diced
2 jalapeño or habanero peppers, diced
1 tbsp fresh or dried rosemary, chopped
1 tbsp fresh or dried thyme, chopped
1 tbsp fresh or dried oregano, chopped
apple cider vinegar to cover
¼–½ cup raw honey

Place the lemon juice and zest, ginger, horseradish, garlic, onion, peppers, rosemary, thyme, and oregano into a quart-size glass jar. Cover with apple cider vinegar, leaving about ½ inch of room at the top. Cover and shake well. Let sit in a cool, dark place for at least 1 month and shake daily.

After 1 month (or longer), use a cheesecloth to strain the vinegar into a clean jar. Squeeze out as much of the vinegar as possible. Add ¼ cup raw honey and stir until fully incorporated. Taste. If you'd like it a little sweeter, add another ¼ cup raw honey and stir again. Feel free to add more honey until you've reached your desired sweetness.

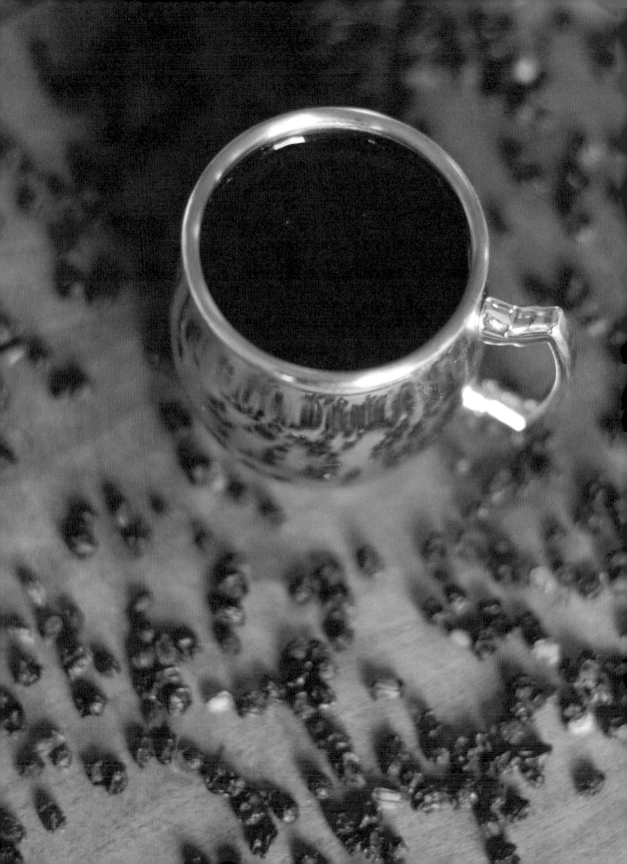

ELDERBERRY IMMUNE BOOST

Yield: 5 cups

If you peek in the medicine cabinet of any wild witch (i.e., herbalist), you'll likely find at least one bottle of elderberry syrup. This ancient classic has been used for thousands of years and is a staple for a very good reason. It is known to be extremely immune boosting and more effective than the flu shot.

Feel free to add other delicious herbs and spices, such as vanilla, cardamom, clove, star anise, and / or orange peel.

3½ cups Medicinal Mushroom Tea (p 5) or filtered water
1 cinnamon stick
1-inch piece fresh ginger root, sliced
⅔ cup dried elderberries
1 cup raw honey
1 cup brandy (optional)*

Put the medicinal mushroom tea in a large saucepan and bring to a boil. Reduce heat to a simmer. Add the cinnamon stick, ginger root, and elderberries. Brew for 20–30 minutes. Strain and add honey; stir until melted. Allow to cool and, if desired, add the brandy. Refrigerate in a sealed container for several weeks.

Brandy helps to preserve this elixir so it will keep for several months, instead of weeks.

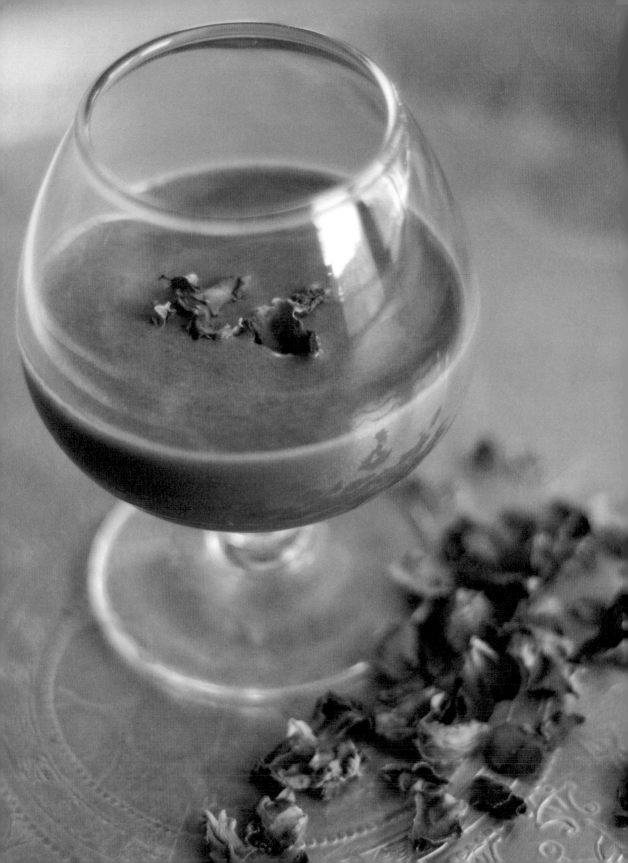

SULTRY SCHISANDRA CHOCOLATE LOVIN'

Yield: 4 ounces; serves 2

A sensually sweet chocolate shot of love made with some favorite herbal aphrodisiacs. Whether you desire a little self-love or want to share an intimate evening with someone special, this shot will definitely get you in the mood. We serve this as an aperitif at my café's annual Valentine's dinner.

Whether you're alone or with your sweetie, I recommend you pick up a Pablo Neruda or Anais Nin book, light some candles, make yourself a bubble bath filled with essential oils and salts, and let the love sink in.

½ cup filtered water
1 tsp schisandra berries
2 tsp damiana leaf
½ cup mylk of choice
6 tbsp raw cacao powder
2 tsp maca powder
2 tsp vanilla extract
2 tbsp raw honey or liquid sweetener of choice

Heat the water in a small saucepan over medium-low heat. Add the schisandra berries and damiana and steep for at least 5 minutes. Strain the tea into a blender and let it cool. Add the mylk, cacao powder, maca powder, vanilla, and honey, then blend for 10–20 seconds, until thoroughly combined. Pour a shot and savor the love.

TIP: If you'd like to extend the magic, feel free to make this as we do most of the other hot elixirs in this book by pouring the shot in a mug and topping off with hot water or your favorite tea.

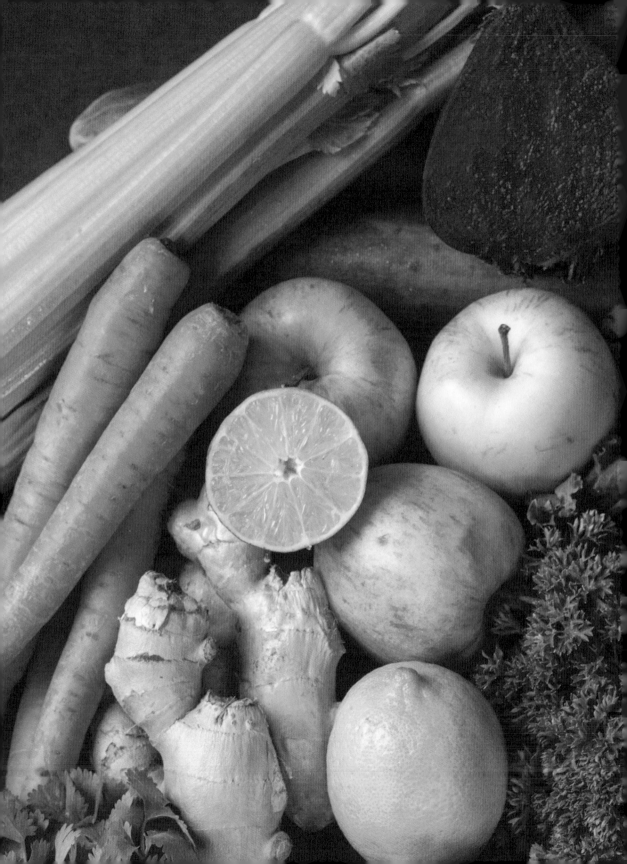

INVIGORATING JUICES

Juices have long been known in the health food world as healing hippie nectars. Once a mysterious liquid found in a hidden, crunchy, patchouli-scented hole in the wall, we are now seeing a steep rise in popularity of high-end juice bars and companies bottling up expensive, cold-pressed brews across the globe.

Once you see how much produce goes into one serving of juice, it's quite impressive to follow that equation through to the amount of vitamins and nutrients delivered in one cup. Since the Standard American Diet is severely lacking in beneficial vitamins and nutrients (in part because of our diet and in part due to depleted soil conditions), increasing our daily intake is crucial to our overall well-being.

Processing your produce through a juicer separates the liquid from the fiber, making it possible to fit a high amount of nutrition into one serving. This is beneficial because without the fiber our bodies are able to assimilate the health benefits very quickly, while expending much less energy than it would take to eat that much produce.

Since most things that offer so much goodness have a dark side, it is important to be careful how much fruit (except citrus) and sweet root (i.e., beet, carrot, sweet potato) juice you consume, as they contain high amounts of sugar. On a regular basis, I personally stick to drinking green juice with very minimal fruit (usually apple, not more than one and ideally green, as green apples are more alkaline than red). The other juices in this book I use as more special occasion drinks instead of my daily go-to.

Juices can be enjoyed as a light snack, an accompaniment to a meal, or as your primary source of nutrition during a cleanse.

Juice cleanses can last as little as one day for a quick reset or as long as 30–60 days, depending on the individual, the circumstances, and the desired results. Traditional juice cleansing is defined as not consuming any fiber, therefore only drinking fresh-pressed or cold-pressed juice and water. Check out my tips in the Nourishing Cleanses chapter (p 187) for more support in preparing for and executing a detox.

TIP: For an extra health boost you can add superfood powders, such as spirulina, chlorella, and camu camu to your juices! Drink your juice right away to reap all the amazing health benefits. Unless cold-pressed and refrigerated, the juice will oxidize, and the nutrients will be lost at a rapid pace.

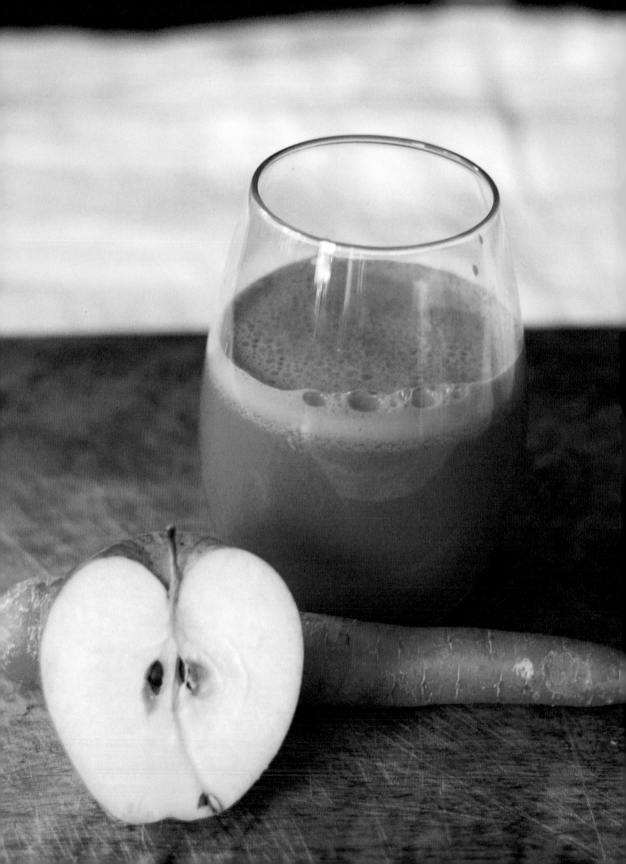

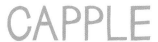

CAPPLE

Yield: 2 cups

A juicing classic, the Capple brings me back to my youth as it is the first fresh-pressed juice I ever remember having. My mom and I would go for walks around the nearly three-mile block we lived on in the summer harvesting Queen Anne's lace, chamomile, and black currants. When we got home she'd pull out the juicer and make Capple juice for us to enjoy as a sweet reward for making it up the steep hill we lived on top of.

5 medium carrots
1 medium apple

Wash, prep, and chop produce as necessary. Process all ingredients through your juicer, alternating between the juicy and more fibrous ingredients. Enjoy!

TIP: When making juice, I like to start processing ingredients like leafy greens, garlic, ginger, and turmeric root near the beginning. You should ALWAYS end with a juicier ingredient, such as a beets, apple, cucumber, or celery. The juicier produce helps wash the more fibrous produce through the juicer, so you don't loose much of its goodness.

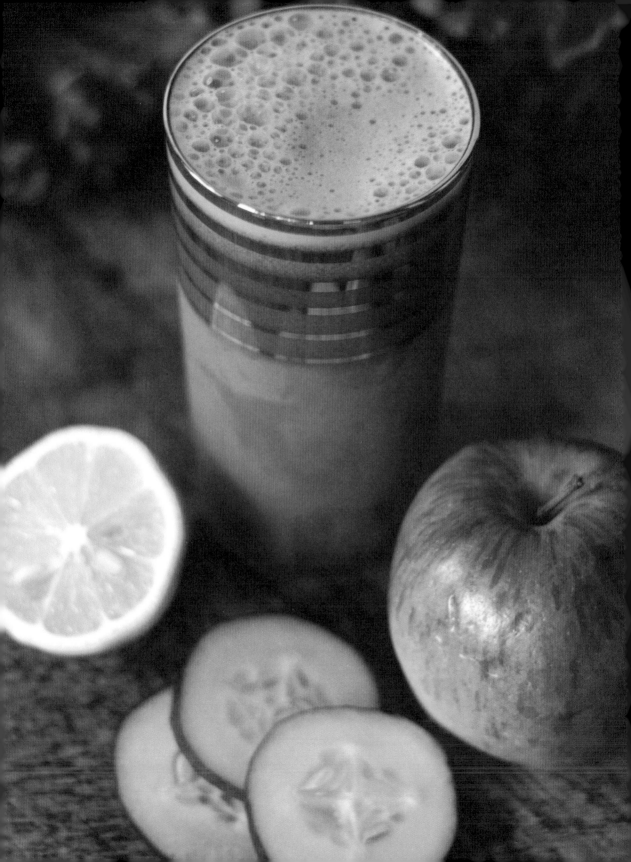

GREEN GODDESS

Yield: 2 cups

Every goddess needs her go-to juice (men, channel that inner divine feminine on this one), and it is in my personal opinion that it should be green. While I occasionally enjoy many of the other juices featured in this book (and beyond), this is hands down my most frequented. Whether I'm looking to start my day off with magical plant-packed energy, am feeling slightly off, or am looking for a midday pick-me-up, this juice never disappoints.

When I'm feeling spicy or under the weather I often add garlic and cayenne for extra immune-boosting goodness.

1 cucumber (skin and all, if organic)
6 celery stalks
1 medium apple
3 leaves of kale (stem and all)
½ lemon (skin and all, if organic)
½-inch sliver of ginger root

SPICE IT UP / MY FAVORITE ADD-ONS (OPTIONAL)
1–3 cloves of garlic (depending on size and personal taste)
pinch of cayenne pepper

Wash, prep, and chop the produce as necessary. Process all ingredients through your juicer, alternating between the juicy and more fibrous ingredients. If adding cayenne, sprinkle on top and whisk in at the end. Enjoy!

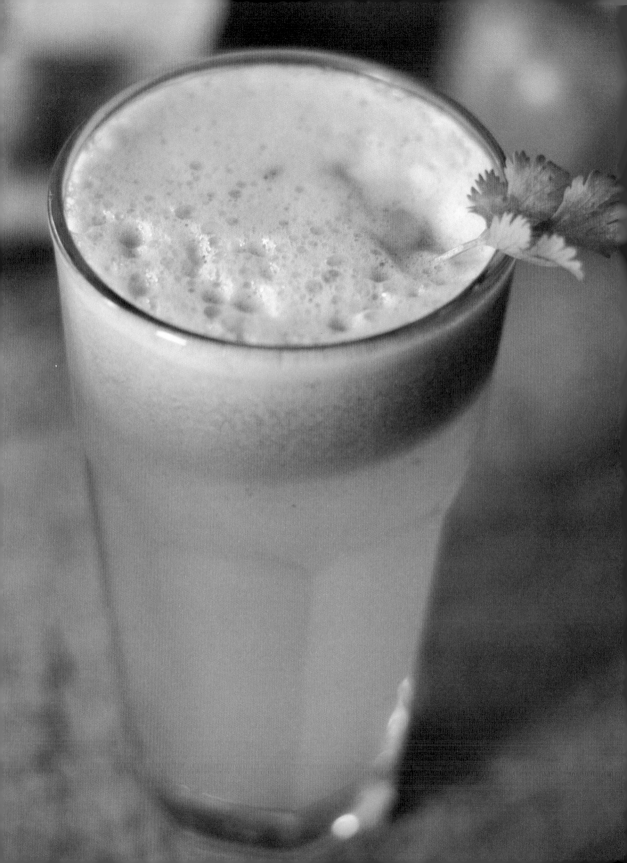

THAI VIBE

Yield: 2 cups

The Thai Vibe is a wonderfully refreshing green juice featuring the powerful cleansing benefits of cilantro, ginger, and lime. Cool down, improve digestion, and flush out heavy metals.

1 cucumber
2 medium apples
¼ lime
¼ bunch cilantro
1-inch chunk ginger

Wash, prep, and chop the produce as necessary. Process all ingredients through your juicer, alternating between the juicy and more fibrous ingredients. Enjoy!

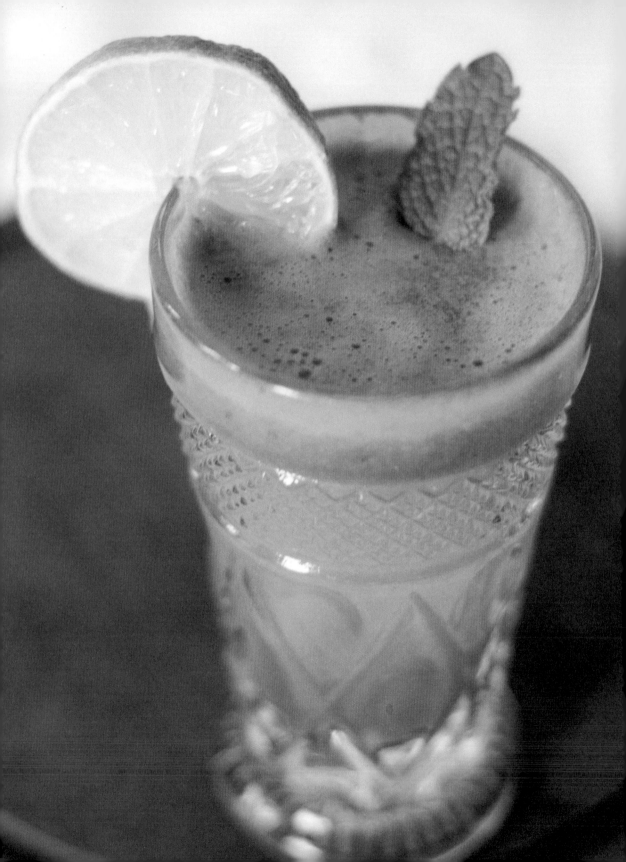

MINT GREEN

Mint Green can be enjoyed year-round, however is best in warmer summer months when you can walk out your back door or down to the farmers' market and gather massive amounts of any kind of mint you can find. Mint eases digestion, reduces inflammation, invigorates energy levels, and cools our bodies, which is such a refreshing feeling during the hotter months.

Perfect in the summer months when mint is in unruly abundance!

4 celery stalks
1 cucumber
1 medium apple
½ lime
3 sprigs mint

Wash, prep, and chop the produce as necessary. Process all ingredients through your juicer, alternating between the juicy and more fibrous ingredients. Enjoy!

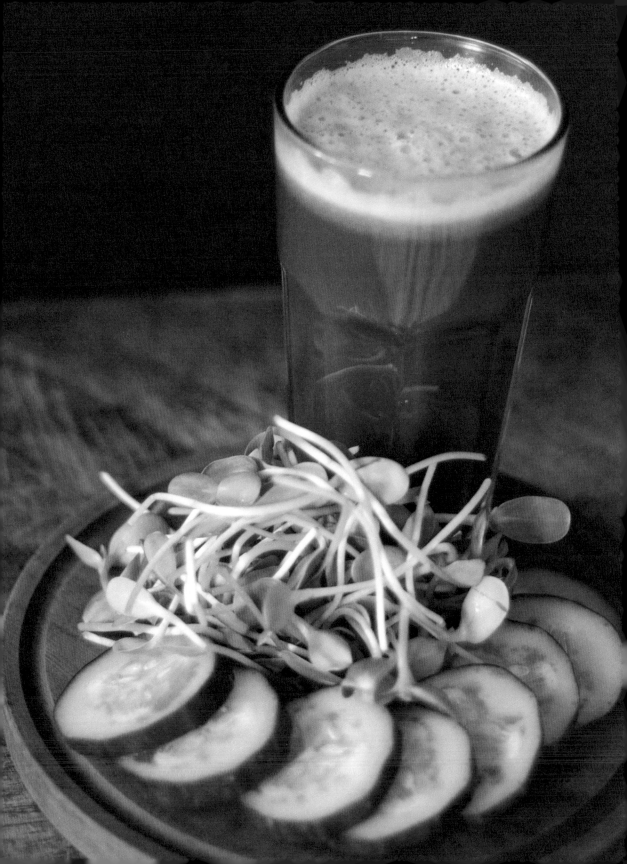

HIPPOCRATES GREEN

Yield: 2 cups

This classic Hippocrates Health Institute-inspired green juice is surprisingly sweet, while remaining sugar-free, since it doesn't include sugary fruits, such as apple, carrot, or beet. If you're on an alkaline cleanse, this is an excellent, healthy addition. While sprouts contain very minimal juice, the vital energy they hold is so powerful because they pack a big punch of vitamins, minerals, and protein, which are all very easily digested. They're also extremely easy to grow at home for year-round greens.

---

large handful of sprouts (pea, sunflower, clover, etc.)
1 cucumber
8 celery stalks

Wash, prep, and chop the produce as necessary. Process all ingredients through your juicer, beginning with the sprouts and ending with the juicier cucumber and celery. Feel the potent life force energy as you drink this one down!

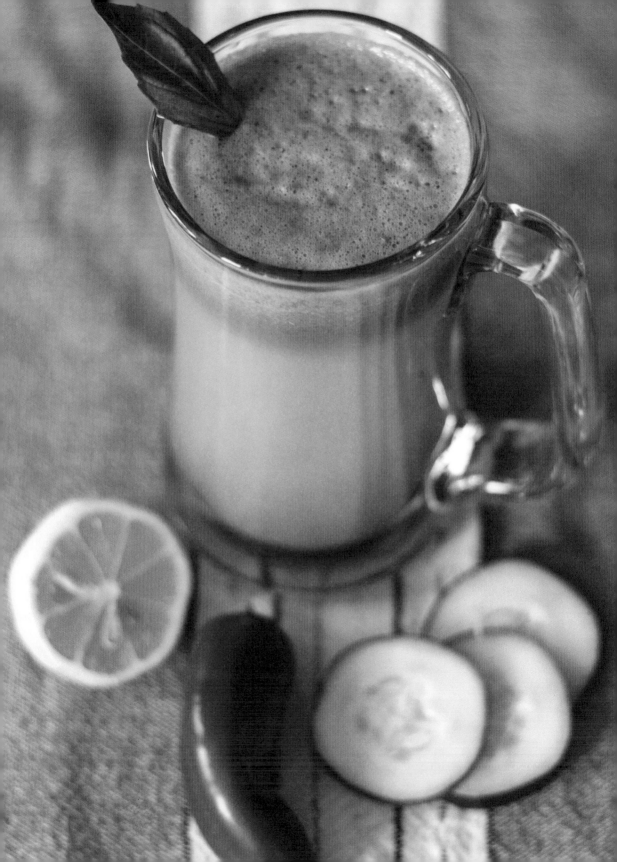

SPICY COOL DOWN

Yield: 2 cups

Cool down and rehydrate with this spicy summer garden-fresh juice.

2 cucumbers
¼ lemon
¼ bunch basil
1–2 jalapeños (depending on personal spice tolerance)

Wash, prep, and chop the produce as necessary. Process all ingredients through your juicer, alternating between the juicy and more fibrous ingredients. Enjoy!

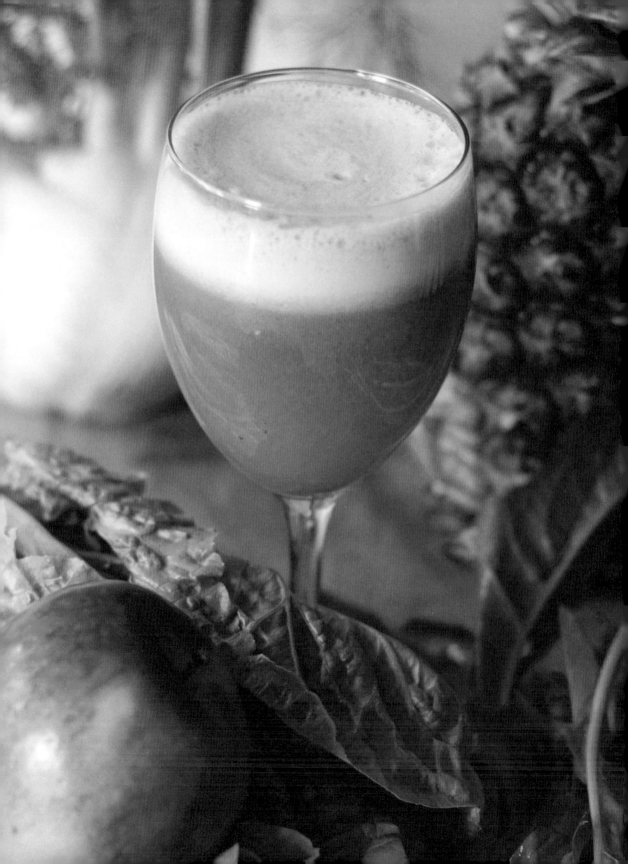

WILD PINE-APPLE FENNEL

Yield: 2 cups

Fresh greens, crisp fruit, and sweet fennel are combined in this soothing elixir for a refreshing, tummy-taming, detoxifying tonic.

In early spring, feel free to walk outside and forage for your own dandelion greens! Make sure to harvest from an area that is free of pesticides and away from the road, and wash before using. While you can still harvest dandelion greens through the fall, they become very bitter and less palatable by late spring into early summer.

1 medium apple
½ pineapple
½ medium fennel bulb
1 head romaine lettuce
½ bunch dandelion greens

Wash, prep, and chop the produce as necessary. Process all ingredients through your juicer, alternating between the juicy and more fibrous ingredients. Enjoy!

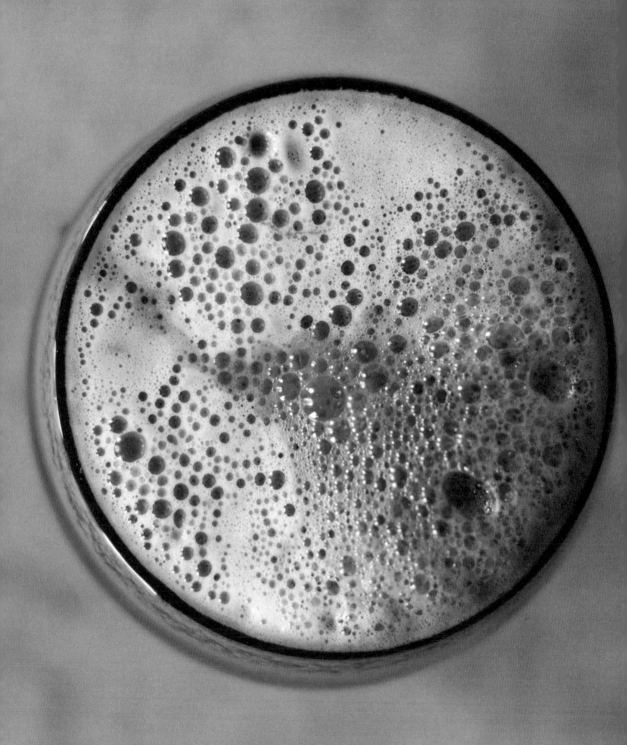

RADIANT RAINBOW

Yield: 2 cups

The aesthetic beauty of this drink is best enjoyed while watching the rainbow of colors flow from your juicer—a beautiful example of plant magic in action!

2 small beets
3 medium carrots
1 medium apple
½-inch sliver of ginger
3 leaves of kale
¼ bunch parsley
¼ lemon

Wash, prep, and chop the produce as necessary. Process all ingredients through your juicer, alternating between the juicy and more fibrous ingredients. Drink the rainbow!

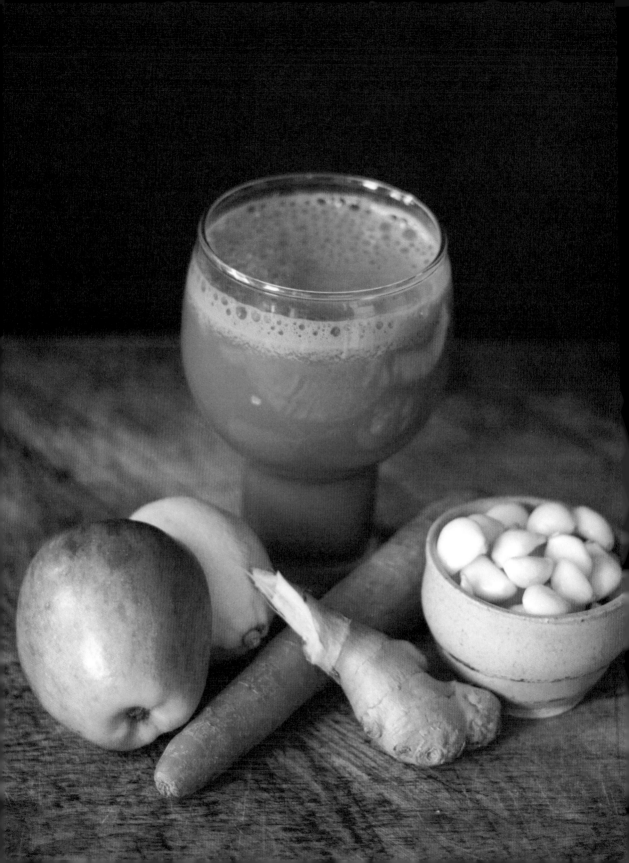

IMMUNITY PROTECTOR

Yield: 2 cups

Perfect as a preventative elixir for cold and flu season or as a healthy jolt when you're feeling under the weather, Immunity juice has you covered with a classic Capple base and added support from some favorite health hero friends: ginger, garlic, lemon, and cayenne.

6 medium carrots
1 apple
½-inch sliver of ginger
3 garlic cloves
½ lemon
⅛ tsp cayenne pepper (optional, for an added boost)

Wash, prep, and chop the produce as necessary. Process all ingredients through your juicer, alternating between the juicy and more fibrous ingredients. If adding cayenne, sprinkle on top and whisk in at the end. Drink to your health!

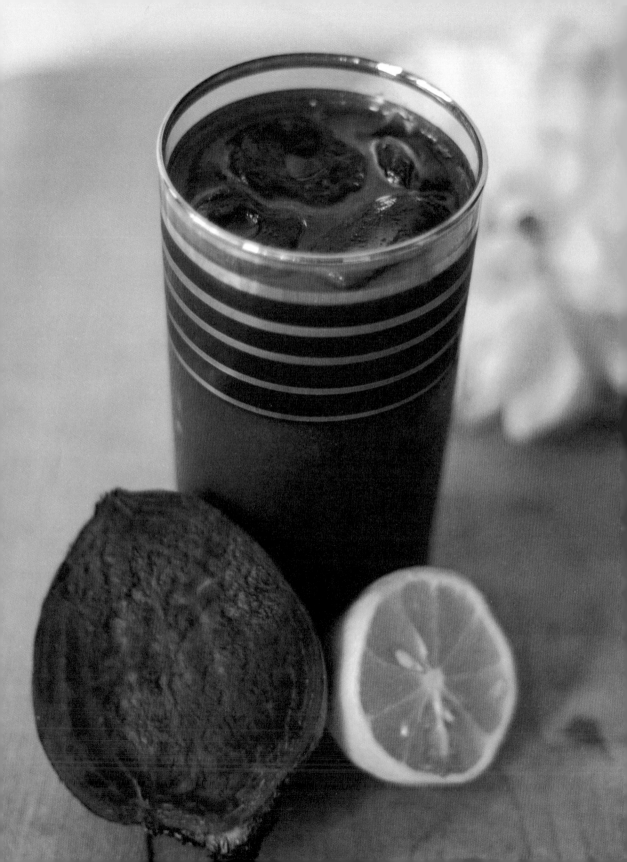

PINK LEMONADE

This pink lemonade is a colorful, fresh-pressed juice twist on everyone's favorite summer staple. Apple is the sweet base liquid, with a little beet added for color, and lemon for that delicious citrus element, keeping this juice true to its name.

2 medium beets
2 medium apples
½ lemon

Wash, prep, and chop the produce as necessary. Process all ingredients through your juicer. Enjoy!

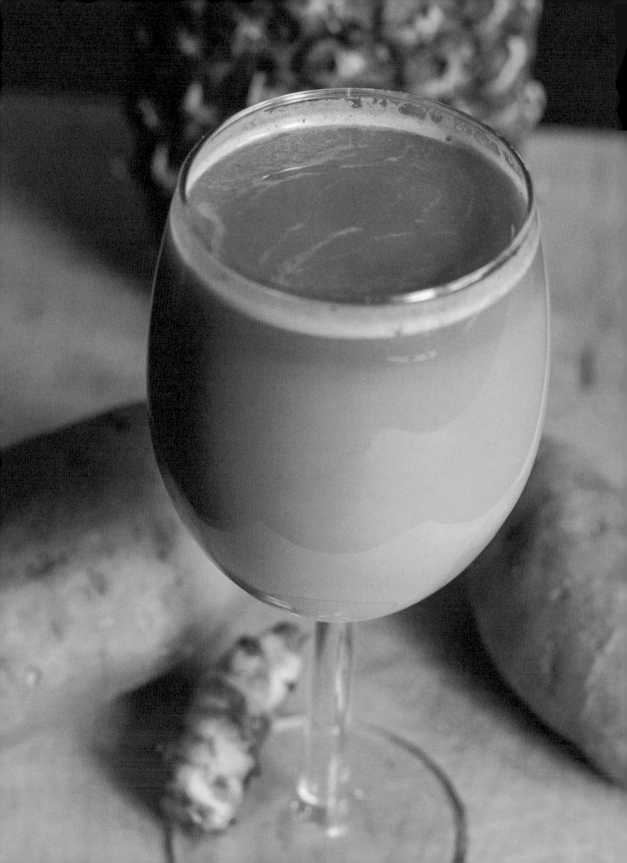

SWEET GOLDEN SUN

Yield: 2 cups

This vibrant juice is packed with so much potent nutrient power. Just thinking about this golden cup of love makes my heart sing and my muscles dance for joy! This blend is a delicious combo filled with anti-inflammatory, energy-boosting, and digestion-soothing properties.

1 inch fresh turmeric root
1 medium sweet potato
½ pineapple

Wash, prep, and chop the produce as necessary. Process all ingredients through your juicer, beginning with the turmeric root to allow the juice of the sweet potato and pineapple to push through the more fibrous root. Sip up and enjoy!

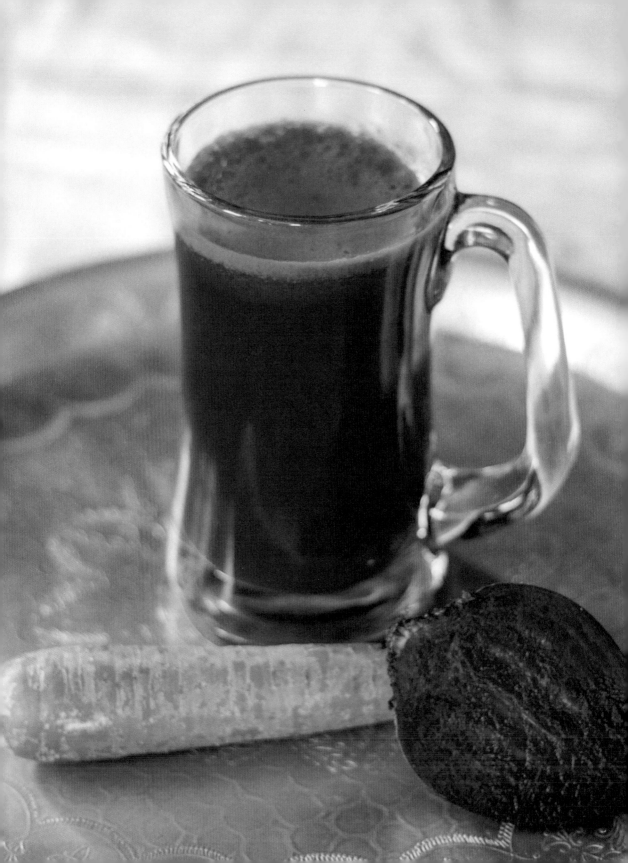

GROUNDING ROOTS

Yield: 2 cups

Sink deep into your root chakra and feel the earthy energy pull you down with this grounding juice.

½-inch sliver of ginger root
2 small beets
4 medium carrots

Wash, prep, and chop the produce as necessary. Process all ingredients through your juicer, beginning with the ginger root to allow the juice of the beets and carrots to push through the more fibrous root. Breathe deep and drink on.

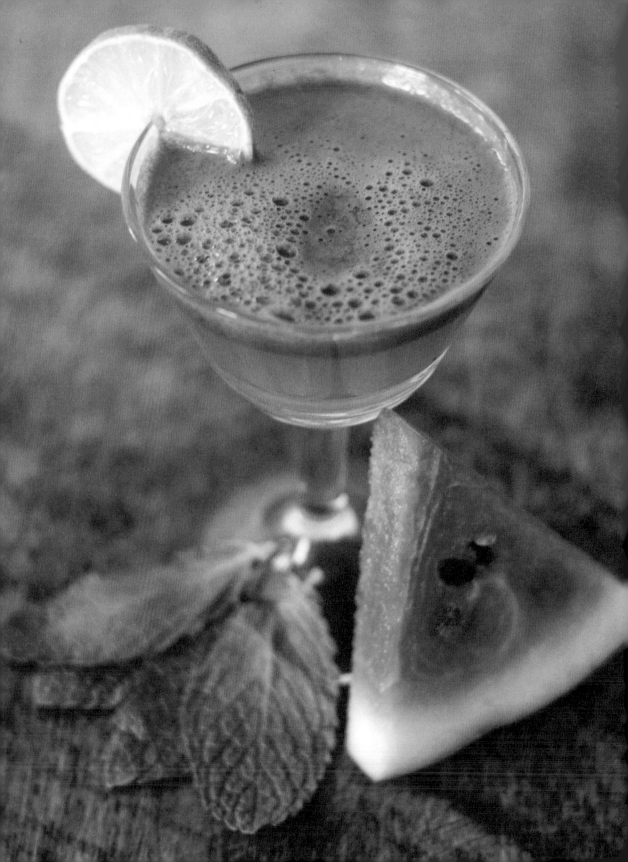

WATERMELON MINT FRESCA

Who doesn't love watermelon in the summer? Combine it with lime and mint and it's quite possibly the most refreshing juice ever—perfect for those unbearably hot, humid summer days made for plunging into cold, secret swimming holes. Super hydrating and wonderfully cooling, you can't go wrong!

¼ watermelon
¼ lime, without the rind
2–3 sprigs of mint

Wash, prep, and chop the produce as necessary. Process all ingredients through your juicer, alternating between the juicy and more fibrous ingredients. Enjoy!

TIP: This makes a great mixer. Try it with Probiotic Ginger Ale (p 183), sparkling water, and / or with your favorite hard alcohol, such as tequila or rum.

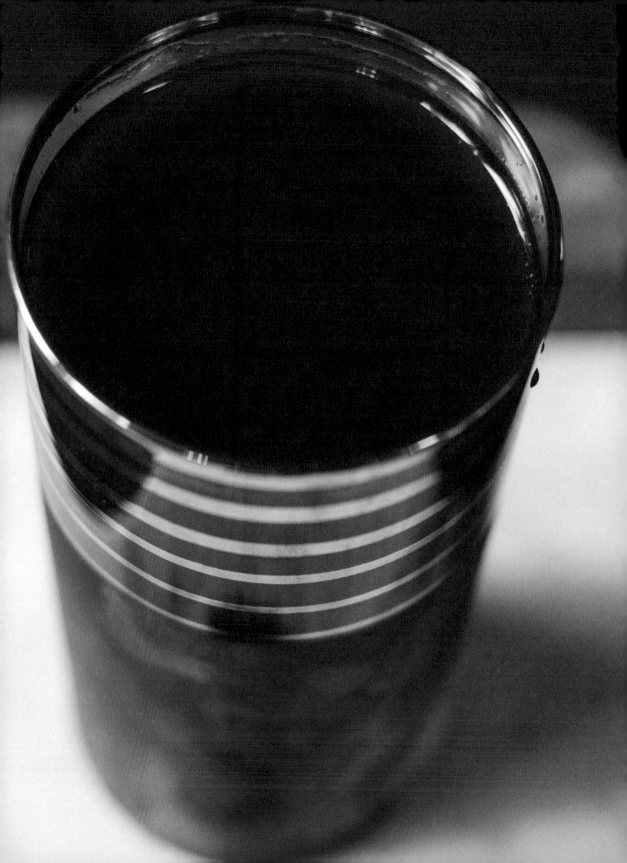

BLACK MAGIC

Yield: 2 cups

This black green juice is extremely cleansing with both apple cider vinegar and the key Black Magic ingredient: activated charcoal, which flushes toxins from the body. While it may sound and / or look completely unappetizing, I promise that once you give it a try you will most likely be swayed; I think this is one of the tastiest juices I've made!

Note: *Do not* use activated charcoal internally if you take any medications, as it flushes everything out of the system. This juice is not intended for everyday use. It is better to drink it once in a while, during a cleanse or while working with your health care practitioner.

1 cucumber
1 medium apple
¼ lemon
½-inch sliver of ginger
2–3 kale leaves
3–5 capsules activated charcoal
1 tbsp apple cider vinegar
filtered water to fill

Wash, prep, and chop the produce as necessary. Process the cucumber, apple, lemon, ginger, and kale through your juicer, alternating between the juicy and more fibrous ingredients.

Pour into a pint-size glass with activated charcoal and apple cider vinegar and whisk together. Fill the glass with filtered water. Sip up and let the toxins go!

TIP: I prefer to use green apples in this recipe, because they're more alkaline, but you can experiment with different apple varieties.

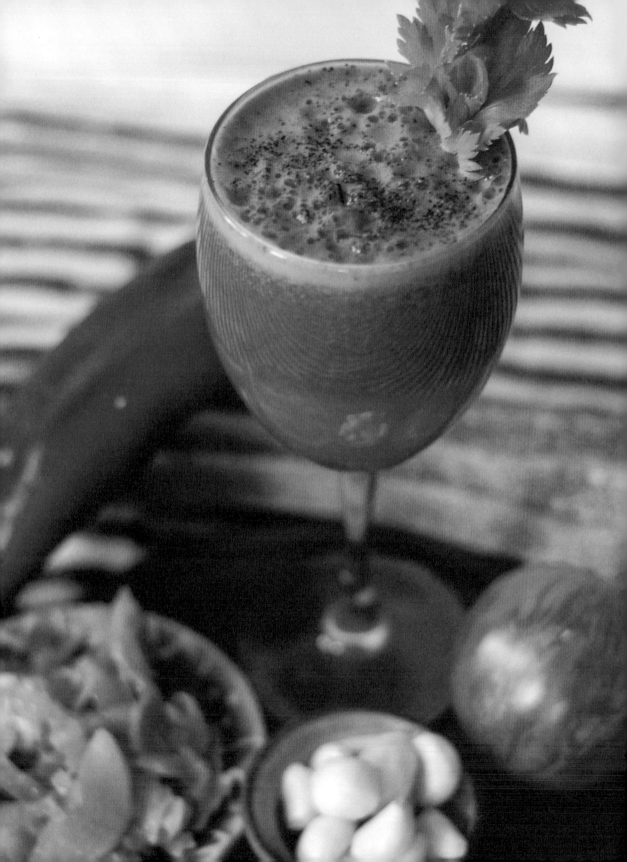

KIMCHI BLOODY MARY

Yield: 2 cups

Have you been throwing out that kimchi brine not knowing what to do with it? Never again, my friend! Food waste ninja to the rescue! I save mine in a jar in the fridge to use for special recipes: kimchi gazpacho, kimchi noodle soup, and Bloody Marys, to name a few. I also just drink straight shots of kimchi brine on occasion . . . don't knock it 'til you've tried it! We make so much kimchi in the Superfresh! kitchen that it stocks up fast. The brine never goes bad and can hang out until you get inspired, although I have a feeling that once you try this drink it might not last that long.

Kimchi is a deliciously addictive (in my very biased opinion) fermented, spicy Korean cabbage condiment that can be found in seemingly endless varieties. It's a great addition to your staple pantry as a yummy side, served with grain, filled into a quesadilla, mixed into fried rice, and so much more.

This is a healthy mocktail, filled with probiotics sure to boost your immunity and enhance your digestion, or killer mixer you can add vodka or saké to. Yes, saké cocktails are delicious!

1 tomato
4-6 celery stalks
½ bell pepper
½ zucchini
¼ lemon

1 clove garlic
¼ cup kimchi brine
⅛ tsp cayenne pepper
    (optional, depending on
    your heat tolerance)
pinch of ground black pepper

Wash, prep, and chop the produce as necessary. Juice the tomato, celery, bell pepper, zucchini, lemon, and garlic, alternating between the juicy and more fibrous ingredients. Mix with the kimchi brine, cayenne, and black pepper. Garnish with a celery stick and enjoy!

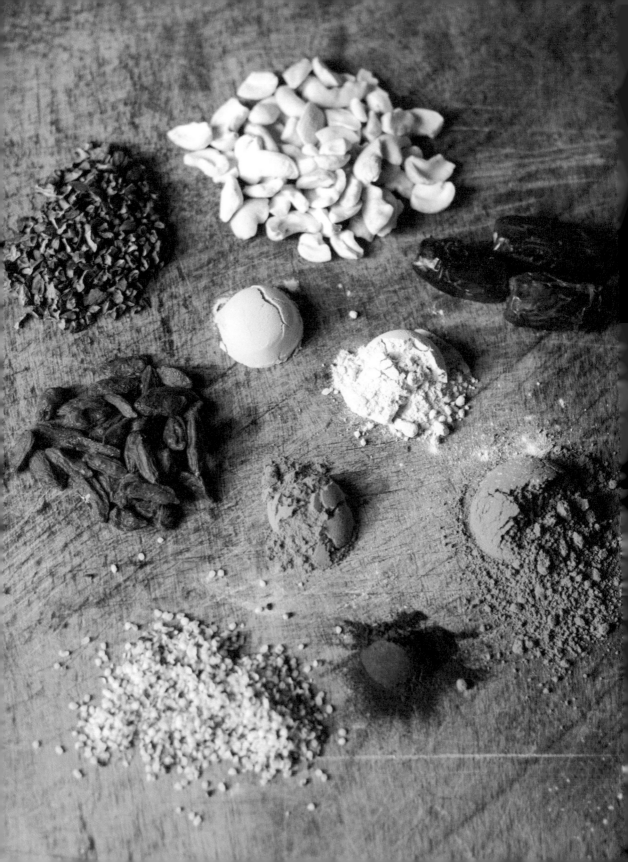

SUPERFOOD SMOOTHIES

Smoothies are the heavier superfood soul sister to juices. Blending everything up breaks down nutrients, making it easier for our bodies to integrate them (versus chewing and expending much more energy), while keeping the fiber-y goodness. Because of this, smoothies are more filling and can serve as a meal because the whole-food content is kept intact.

These blends are the perfect vehicles for delivering many of your favorite supplements / superfoods into the sacred temple of your glorious body. I go on and off with daily smoothie consumption, as well as following a strict supplement regimen. However, when I'm on my A game with both, I throw in literally everything I want to make sure I get a daily dosage into one big crazy blend (including, but not limited to: coconut oil, plant-based omega 3-6-9 oil, bee pollen, chia seeds, super-green powders, hemp seeds, etc.). Pick your favorite smoothie base and add in whatever your heart—and body—desires! Check out the Custom Superfood Add-On Guide (p 232) for helpful measurements when building your own concoction.

When I did my first juice cleanse, which lasted for 14 days, the thing I was most concerned about was not consuming any fiber. To ease myself into this cleanse I decided to include smoothies in my diet; I just didn't add any sweeteners. Two of my favorites from my beloved café are the Green Giant (p 127) and the Funky Monkey (p 129).

While my body is able to handle the sugar content in smoothies a bit better than juices due to the inclusion of fiber, I do try to minimize my fruit intake here as well. One summer I consumed far too many berries, primarily in smoothie form, which resulted in an adverse health reaction, and I had to completely eliminate all fruit for months in order to recover. I also learned a very important lesson of mixing things up every once in a while; for instance, I normally go for hemp mylk, but try to take breaks from it once in a while and switch to a different type of mylk. This same logic can be applied to foods, superfoods, and herbs in any form, as overconsumption can lead to the development of food intolerances or allergies, a decrease or plateau in benefits, or other negative health impacts.

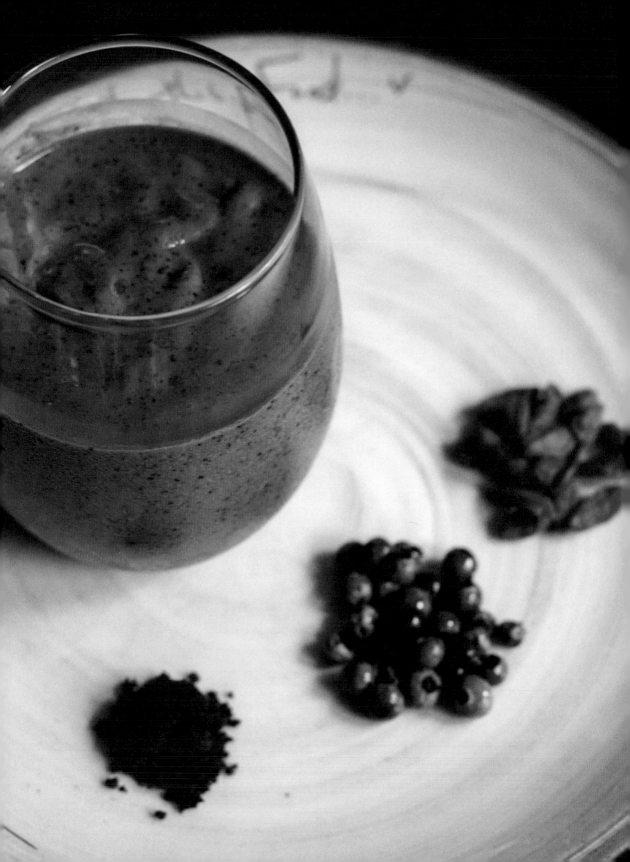

SUPERBERRY DREAM

Yield: 2 cups

One of the most popular smoothies we serve, the Superberry Dream is so berry-licious and jam-packed with antioxidants that it will likely become your favorite go-to berry smoothie! We take the quintessential berry smoothie and add goji berries and acai powder for an added superfood boost.

1 cup mylk of choice
1 frozen banana
½ cup frozen strawberries
½ cup frozen blueberries
1 tbsp goji berries
1 tsp acai powder
2 tbsp Date Paste (p 25)

Blend all ingredients together until super smooth. Enjoy the sweet berry goodness.

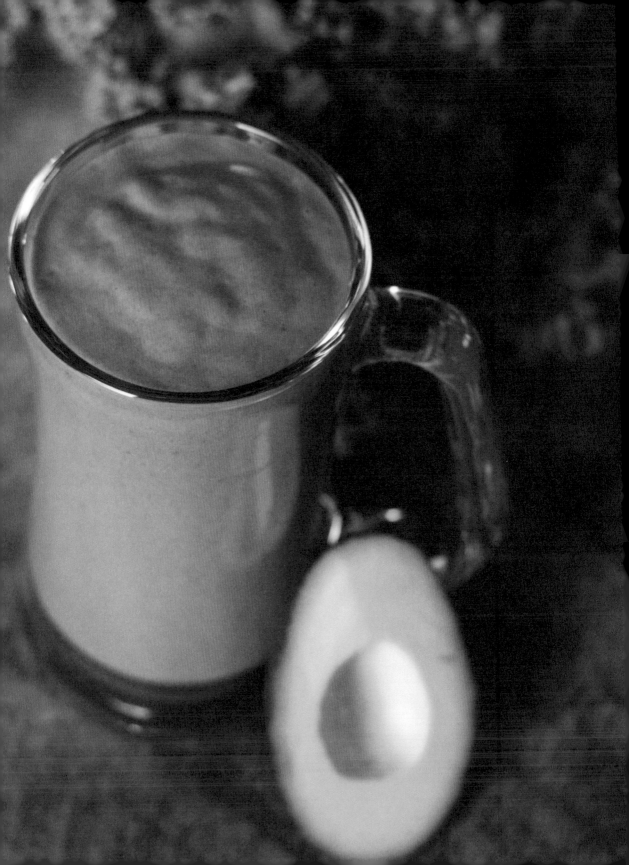

GREEN GIANT

Yield: 2 cups

The ultimate green smoothie made for the Hulk in us all. Avocado adds a silky, thick creaminess, along with extra-filling healthy fat. Every green smoothie needs a dark leafy green, and I'm partial to kale.

To make it extra dark green and to include next-level nutrient-rich superfoods, the Green Giant adds two popular powerhouse blue-green algaes: spirulina and chlorella.

===

1 cup mylk of choice
1½ frozen bananas
¼ tsp spirulina
¼ tsp chlorella
2–3 kale leaves
¼ avocado
½ tsp vanilla extract
1-inch slice fresh ginger root

===

Blend all ingredients together until super smooth. Feel the power of the greens in each sip!

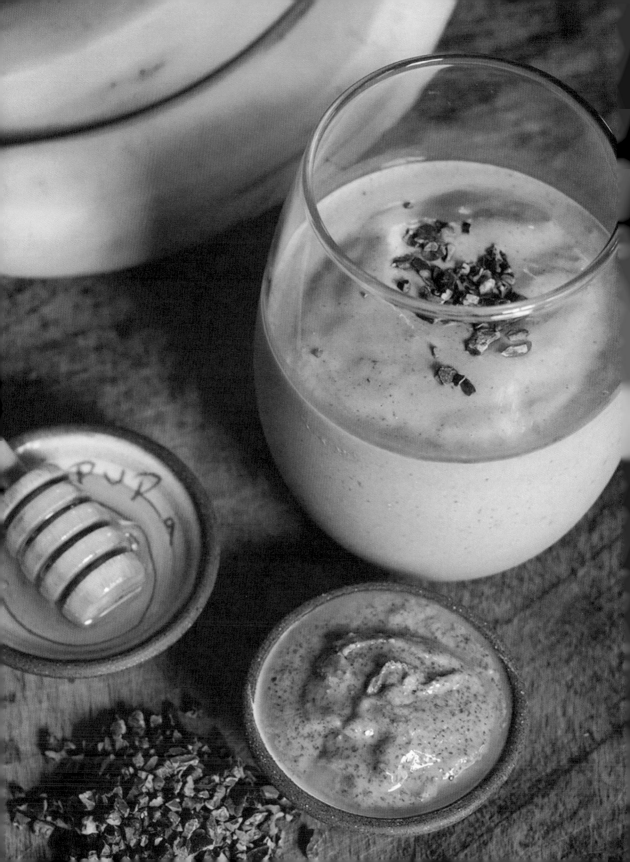

FUNKY MONKEY

Yield: 2 cups

You can never go wrong with the tried-and-true combo of nut butter, banana, and chocolate. Superfresh! has a peanut-free kitchen, so we use almond butter in our recipe. This is one of my most frequently consumed smoothies and it is always satisfying. Always.

I remember the first health food restaurant I went to. My mom would take me there after my gymnastics class when I was around nine years old. We didn't go often, but I always got the rice mylk, peanut butter, banana, chocolate smoothie. It was easily my childhood favorite, having the power to instantly make me happy.

1 cup mylk of choice
1½ frozen bananas
1 tbsp raw cacao powder
2 tbsp almond butter
1 tbsp raw honey or liquid sweetener of choice
1 tbsp raw cacao nibs

Blend together the mylk, bananas, cacao powder, almond butter, and honey until super smooth. Add the cacao nibs and blend for another 10 seconds or so—you want them to remain slightly crunchy. Try not to get a brain freeze!

TIP: Add 1 tbsp maca powder and / or half the mylk and add ½ cup Cold Brew Concentrate (p 33) for a "Spunky Monkey!"

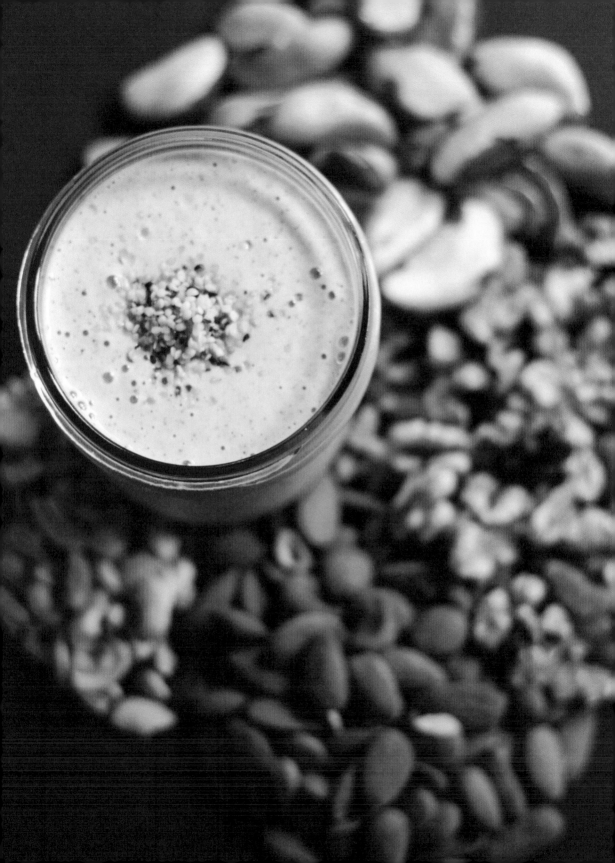

NUT MEISTER

Yield: 2 cups

This smoothie recipe came about in response to a friend's request for a thick and nutty frozen blend. It's filled with four different kinds of nuts, plus hemp seeds for good measure and an added protein kick. Extremely filling and perfect before or after a big workout.

1 cup mylk of choice
1 frozen banana
1 tbsp almond butter
¼ cup cashews
¼ cup brazil nuts
¼ cup walnuts
1 tbsp hemp seeds
2 tbsp pure maple syrup

Blend together all ingredients until super smooth. Drink it in pre- or post-workout.

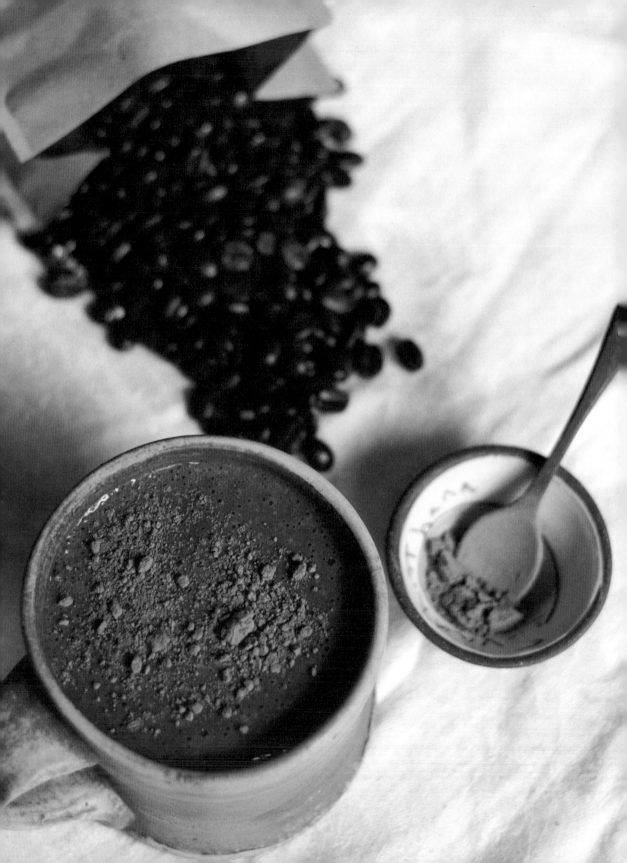

MOCHA DREAM

If you love caffeine and chocolate, this is the smoothie for you! Cold brew concentrate is deceptively strong and so insanely delicious; this will definitely hype you up!

¼ cup mylk of choice
¾ cup Cold Brew Coffee (p 33)
2 frozen bananas
3 tbsp raw cacao powder
½ tsp vanilla extract
1 tbsp pure maple syrup
3–4 ice cubes
dash of cinnamon

Blend all ingredients together until super smooth. Fly high on the super energy boost!

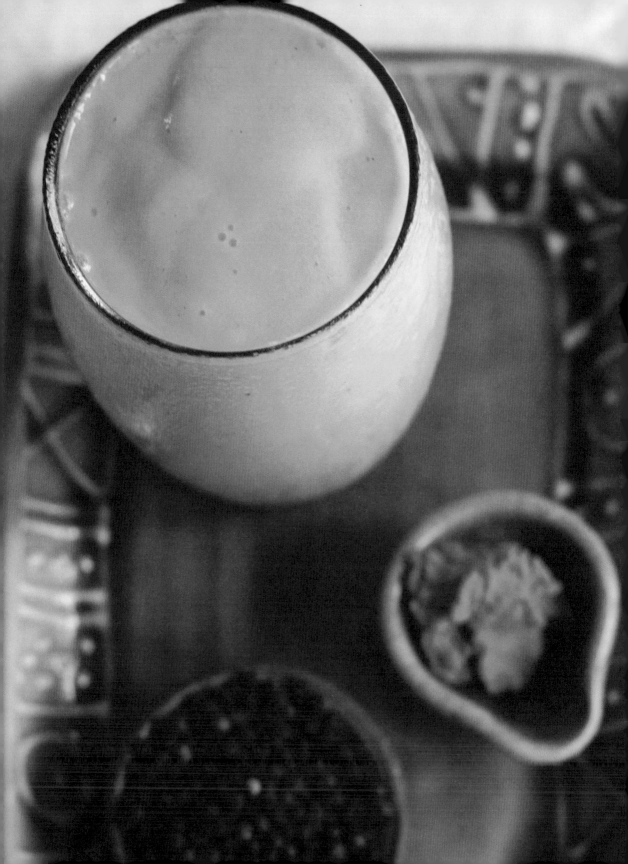

GOLDEN GODDESS

Yield: 2 cups

This smoothie is essentially Golden Mylk meets a mango lassi for a yummy Indian-inspired frozen treat that is both cooling and anti-inflammatory!

1 cup coconut mylk
1 cup frozen mango
1 tsp Turmeric Paste (p 23)
½-inch sliver of ginger
½ tsp vanilla extract
1 tbsp Date Paste (p 25)

Blend together all ingredients until super smooth. Enjoy!

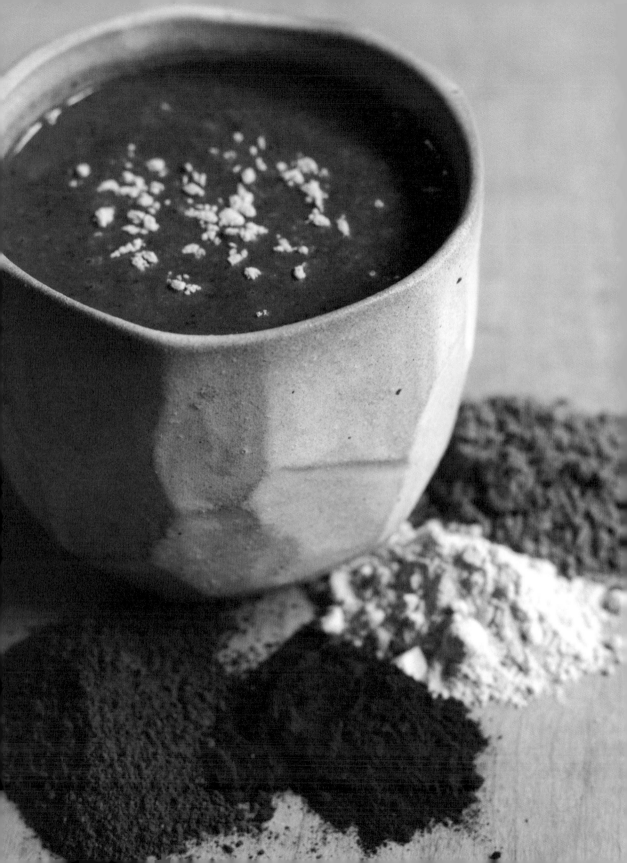

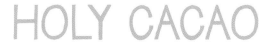

HOLY CACAO

One of my all-time favorite smoothies, this recipe combines so many of my favorite things into one insanely flavorful frozen cup of love!

The word cacao is derived from the Mayan word *ka'kau'*. It was a drink of the Mayan gods, and the beans were used as currency, often hollowed out as counterfeit. The serving of cacao in this smoothie is considered a ceremonial dosage. Don't worry, while it is in fact a stimulant, cacao is not actually caffeinated.

Combining such a sacred superfood with the King of Medicinal Mushrooms (chaga), an Ayurvedic staple (holy basil), and a much-coveted Peruvian Powerhouse (maca) makes for a very holy healing drink indeed. It should be something you slowly savor, but I have to admit, mine always disappears so much faster than any other smoothie.

1 cup Mylk (p 21)
3 tbsp raw cacao powder
½ tsp chaga powder
1 tsp maca powder
⅛ tsp holy basil extract powder
1 frozen banana
½ cup frozen blueberries (raspberries are also crazy delicious!)
2 tbsp Date Paste (p 25) or liquid sweetener of choice (optional)

Blend all ingredients together until super smooth. Savor all the sacred goodness.

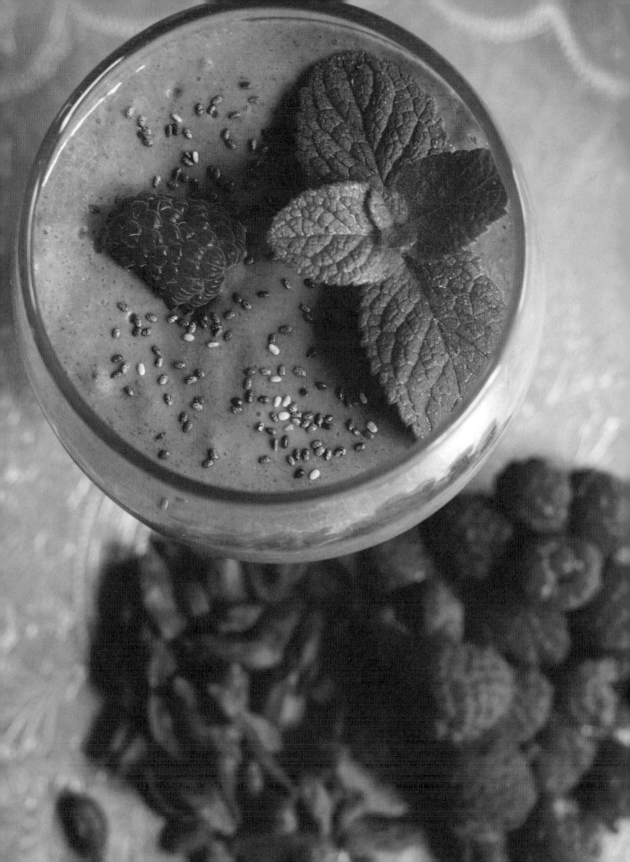

CHI-GOJI-LICIOUS

Yield: 2 cups

Sweet, tart, and powerful, this is my personal favorite berry smoothie. Less sweet than the Superberry Dream, and extra energy boosting with chia seeds and goji berries, this truly is chi-goji-licious!

1 cup mylk of choice
1 frozen banana
½ cup frozen raspberries
1 tbsp chia seeds
1 tbsp goji berries
2 tbsp Date Paste (p 25)

Blend all ingredients together until super smooth. Enjoy!

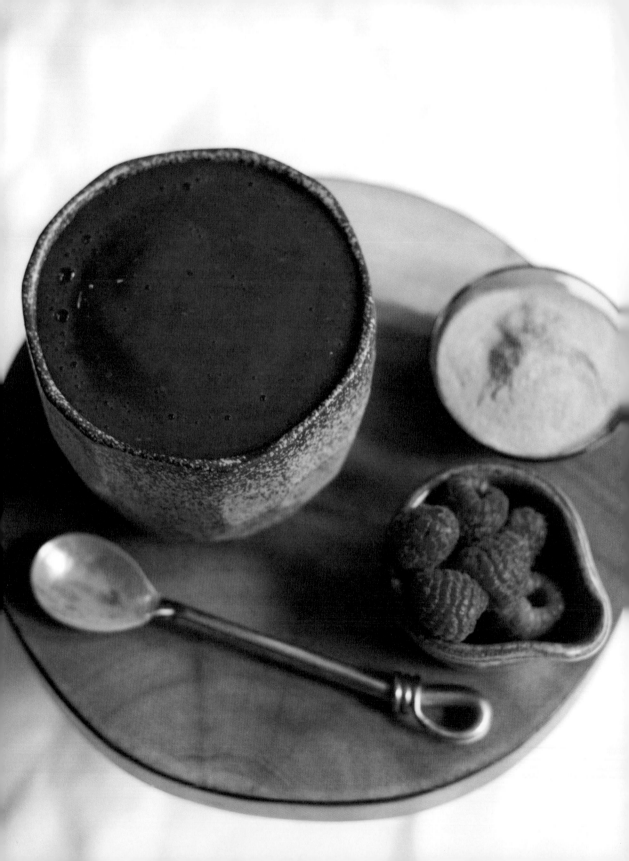

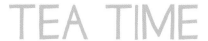

TEA TIME

Yield: 2 cups

With a double dose of green tea goodness, Tea Time delivers a clean, energizing caffeine boost and loads of antioxidants. Blended with frozen raspberries and a little banana, this is essentially a raspberry green tea sorbet. Yum!

1 cup iced green tea
1 cup frozen raspberries
1 tbsp Date Paste (p 25) or liquid sweetener of choice
1 tsp matcha green tea powder

Blend all ingredients together until super smooth. Drink this one slowly to keep brain freeze at bay.

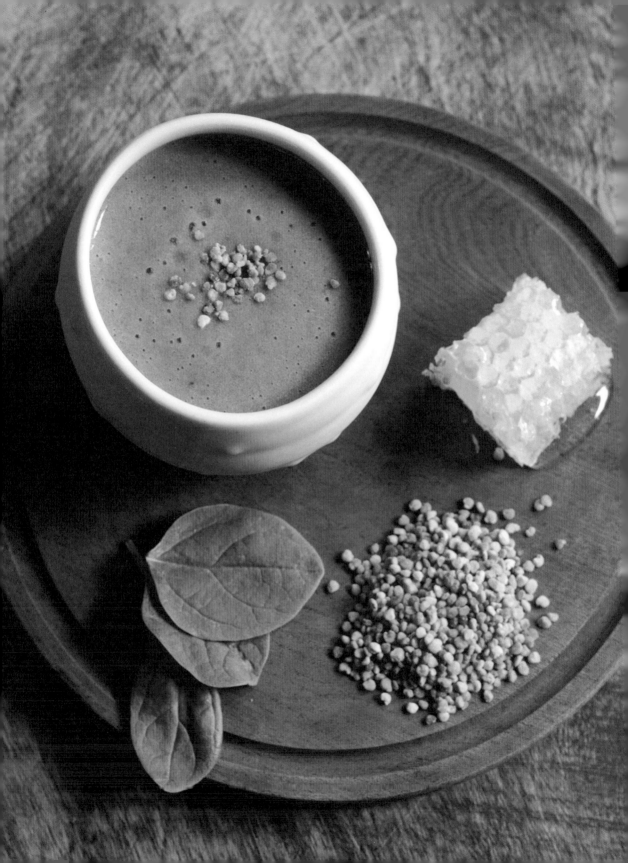

BEE LOVE

Yield: 2 cups

Sweet, light, green, and refreshing. This is happiness in smoothie form. Think frolicking in fields of wildflowers with clear blue skies above or hanging at the beach with good friends. Enjoy year-round for a taste of summer!

1 cup pineapple juice
1½ frozen bananas
1 cup spinach
1 tbsp raw honey
1 tbsp bee pollen (optional)

Blend all ingredients together until super smooth. Sip up the summertime vibe!

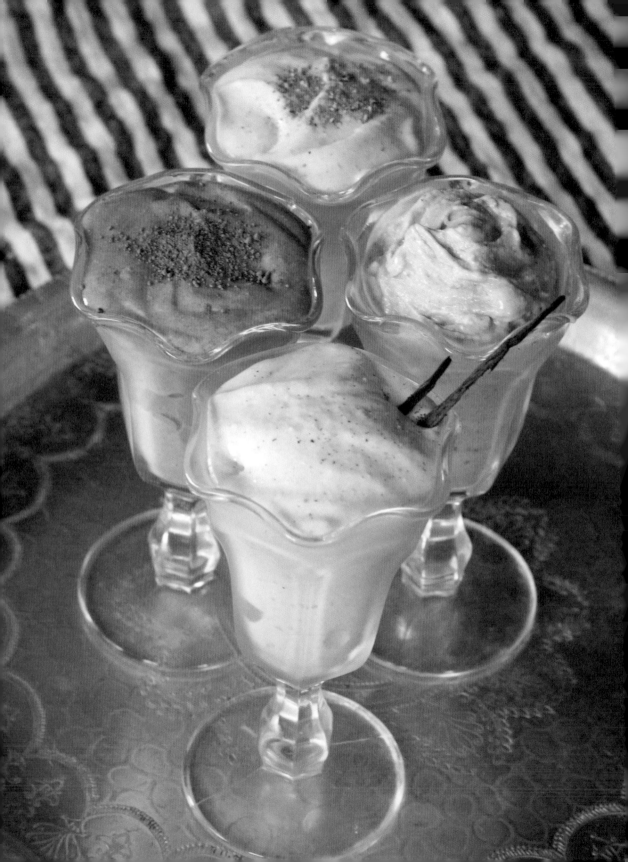

MYLKSHAKES

Who doesn't love a good, thick mylkshake? We've got your classics covered and offer a chai variation for a warming, spicy twist.

VANILLA
1 cup mylk of choice
1½ frozen bananas
1 tbsp vanilla extract
2 tbsp Date Paste (p 25)
¼ cup raw cashew pieces
several pieces of ice

STRAWBERRY
1 cup mylk of choice
1 frozen banana
⅓ cup frozen strawberries
1 tsp vanilla extract
2 tbsp Date Paste (p 25)
¼ cup raw cashew pieces
several pieces of ice

CHOCOLATE
1 cup mylk of choice
1½ frozen bananas
1 tsp vanilla extract
2 tbsp raw cacao powder
2 tbsp Date Paste (p 25)
¼ cup raw cashew pieces
several pieces of ice

CHAI
1 cup mylk of choice
1½ frozen bananas
1 tsp vanilla extract
2 tbsp Date Paste (p 25)
¼ cup raw cashew pieces
2 tsp chai spice mix
1 tsp ginger juice
several pieces of ice

Choose your desired flavor. Blend all ingredients together until super smooth. Let yourself be transported to your childhood happy place!

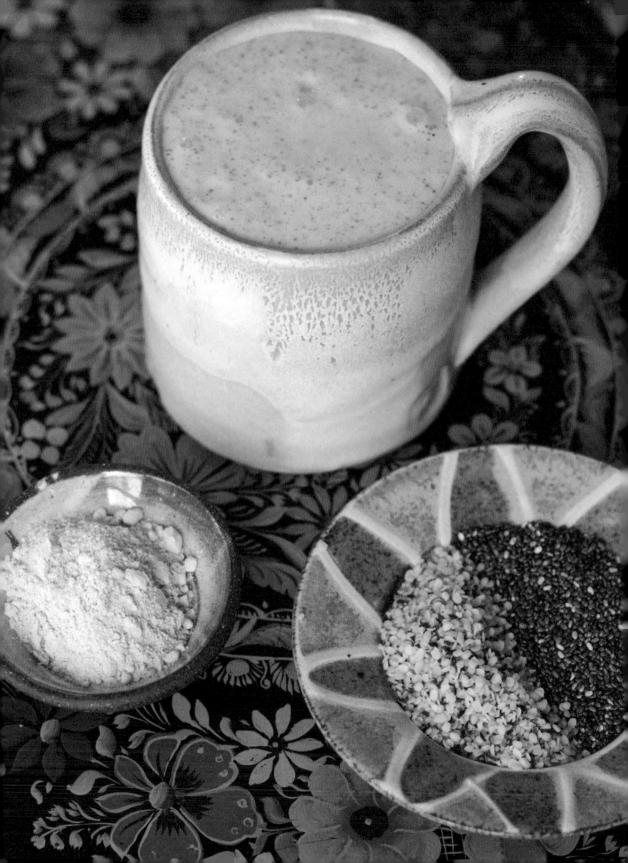

MARVELOUS MACA

Yield: 2 cups

One of the most delicious and underappreciated smoothies we offer at the café, the Marvelous Maca is filled with so much goodness: adaptogenic / aphrodisiac maca and my two favorite super seeds, chia and hemp. Protein rich, balancing, energizing—this smoothie packs a great punch of power!

1 cup mylk of choice
1½ frozen bananas
1 tbsp maca powder
1 tbsp hemp seeds
1 tbsp chia seeds
1 tsp vanilla extract
2 tbsp Date Paste (p 25)

Blend all ingredients together until super smooth. Try to savor all the sacred goodness.

TIP: Due to the flavor profile of this drink it is a wonderful base for throwing in your favorite add-ons. I like to add spirulina, raw cacao powder, or almond butter.

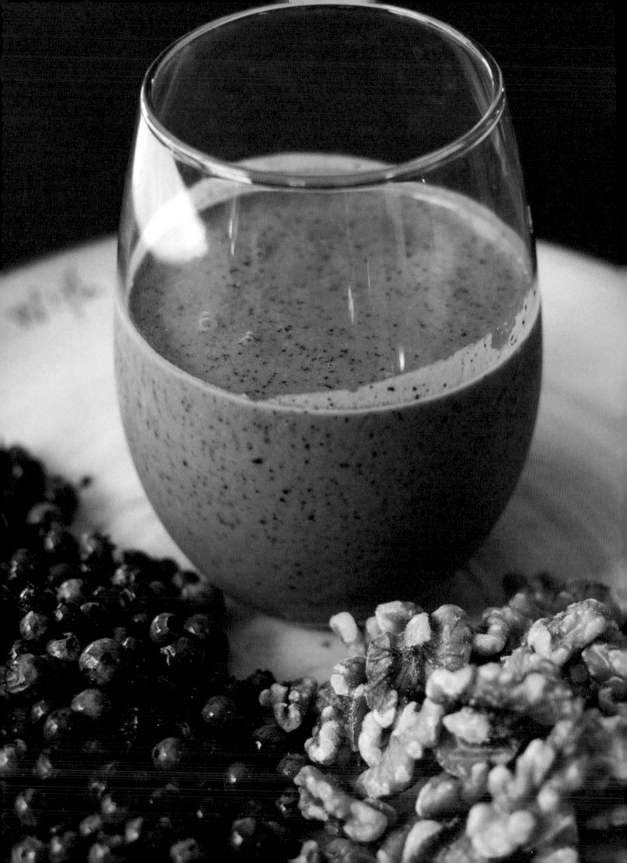

PURPLE PASHA

Magical maca mixed with wild blueberries, walnuts, and coconut water make this a vibrant deep purple cup made for the cosmos.

1 cup coconut water
1 frozen banana
½ cup frozen blueberries
1 tsp maca powder
¼ cup walnuts
2 tbsp Date Paste (p 25)
½ tsp vanilla extract
several pieces of ice

Blend all ingredients together until super smooth. Channel the purple power as you drink this down.

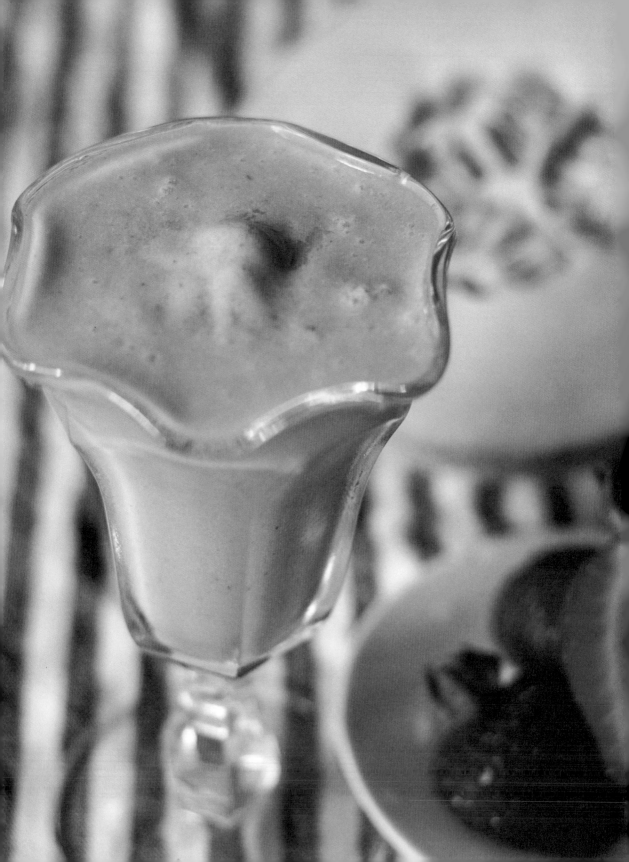

BERRY MELON BLISS

Yield: 2 cups

One day at the café, we received an email from one of our farmers saying that the farm had an amazing crop of cantaloupe with a link to cantaloupe smoothie recipes we could feature this delicious melon in if we loaded up and ordered 40 pounds. We took the melons, accepted the challenge, and I woke up a few days later dreaming of the flavor combo of cantaloupe and lucuma with some strawberries thrown in for good measure! The rest is delicious history.

1 cup mylk of choice
½ cup frozen cantaloupe
1 cup frozen strawberries
1 tsp lucuma
2 tbsp Date Paste (p 25)

Blend all ingredients together until super smooth. Bliss out with this sweet melon-y goodness!

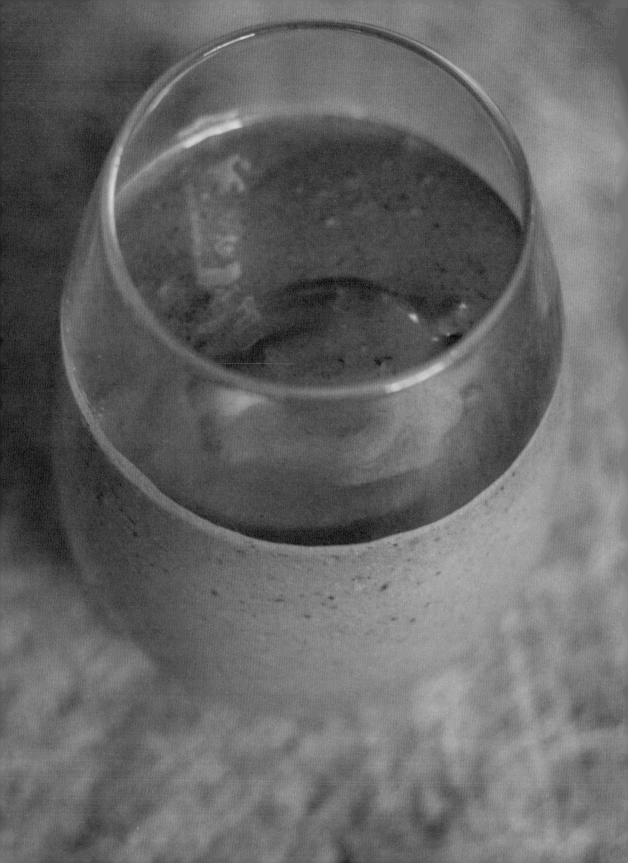

CHOCOLATE CHERRY CHEEZECAKE

Yield: 2 cups

I think the name of this smoothie says it all. This is pure luxury in smoothie form.

1 cup coconut mylk
½ cup frozen cherries
1 frozen banana
¼ cup raw cashew pieces
2 tbsp raw cacao powder
½ tsp vanilla extract
pinch of Himalayan salt
2 tbsp pure maple syrup

Blend all ingredients together until super smooth. Drink in the velvety goodness.

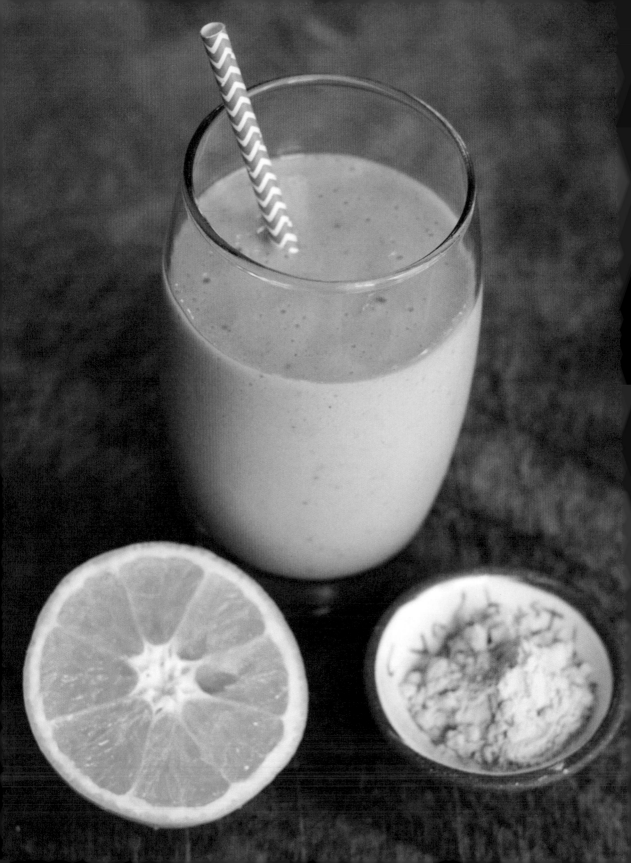

ORANGE DREAMSICLE

Yield: 2 cups

This definitely harkens back to a flavor of my childhood. Popsicles, frozen creamy orange drinks, and summer fun! Between orange juice and camu camu, this drink is slam packed with a great dose of vitamin C to boost your immune system!

½ cup orange juice
½ cup coconut mylk
1½ frozen bananas
¼ cup raw cashew pieces
1 tsp camu camu powder
½ tsp vanilla extract
2 tbsp Date Paste (p 25)

Blend all ingredients together until super smooth, then drink up the creamy orange deliciousness!

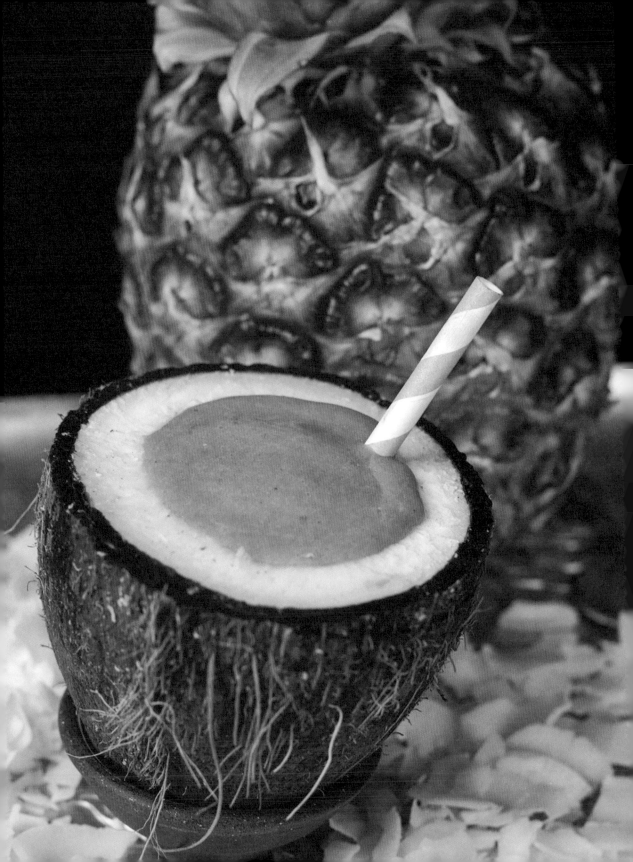

SWEET GREEN PIÑA COLADA

Yield: 2 cups

This beach-time classic is infused with some next-level green magic with the addition of spinach and moringa powder. It may quickly become your new favorite happy hour smoothie. Just remember, it's always happy hour somewhere!

⅓ cup coconut mylk
⅔ cup pineapple juice
1½ frozen bananas
1 cup spinach
1 tsp moringa powder
2 tbsp Date Paste (p 25)

Blend all ingredients together until super smooth. Dig your toes into the sand and revel in the goodness!

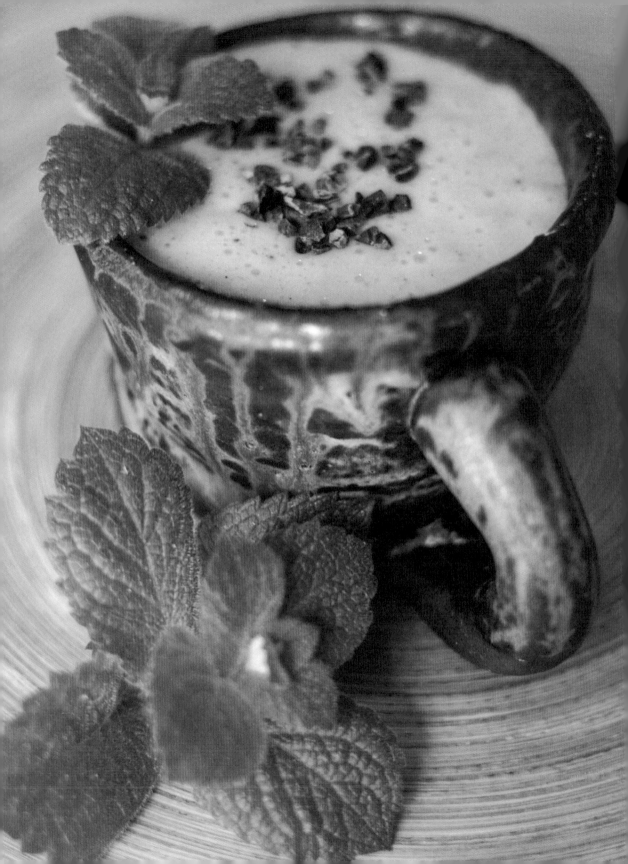

MYSTICAL MINT

Yield: 2 cups

A classic combination, Mystical Mint may transport you to far-off intergalactic places made in your dreams of billowy clouds, stars, and supernovas.

1 cup mylk of choice
1½ frozen bananas
½ tsp peppermint extract
1 tsp lucuma powder
1 tbsp cacao nibs
several pieces of ice

Blend all ingredients together until super smooth. Drink up the magic!

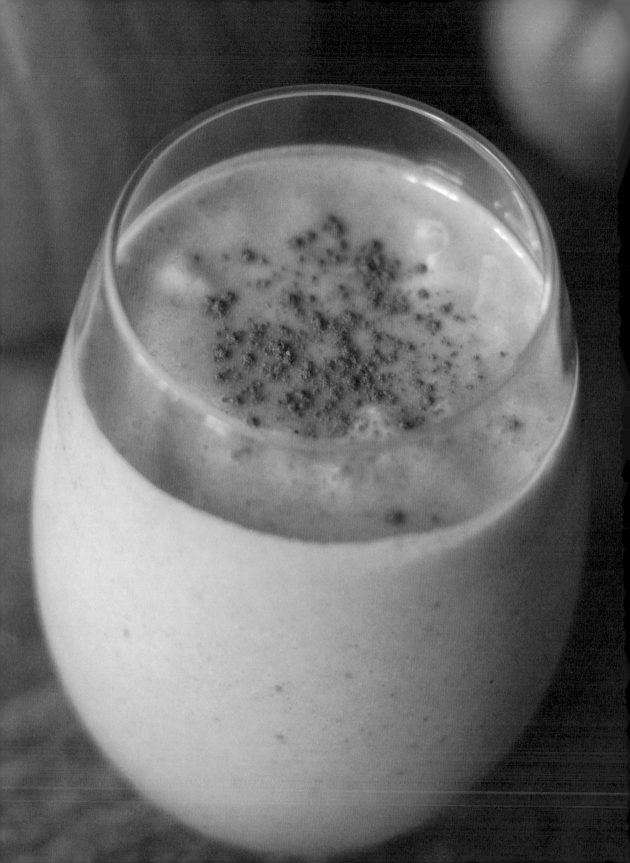

PUMPKIN PIE

Yield: 2 cups

I know that as soon as September hits, *everything* turns to pumpkin this and squash that, but for very good reason—winter squash is *oh so* delicious and crazy abundant! Wrap up in lots of cozy layers and welcome autumn's crisp air, crunchy leaves, and breathtaking foliage.

This Pumpkin Pie smoothie tastes like a frozen version of creamy, silky smooth pumpkin pie filling. How can you resist?!

1 cup mylk of choice
1 frozen banana
½ cup pumpkin puree
1 tsp cinnamon
¼ tsp nutmeg
½-inch sliver of fresh ginger root
1 tsp maca powder
1 tsp vanilla extract
2 tbsp Date Paste (p 25)

Blend all ingredients together until super smooth. Enjoy for the handful of months it is acceptable to indulge in all things pumpkin!

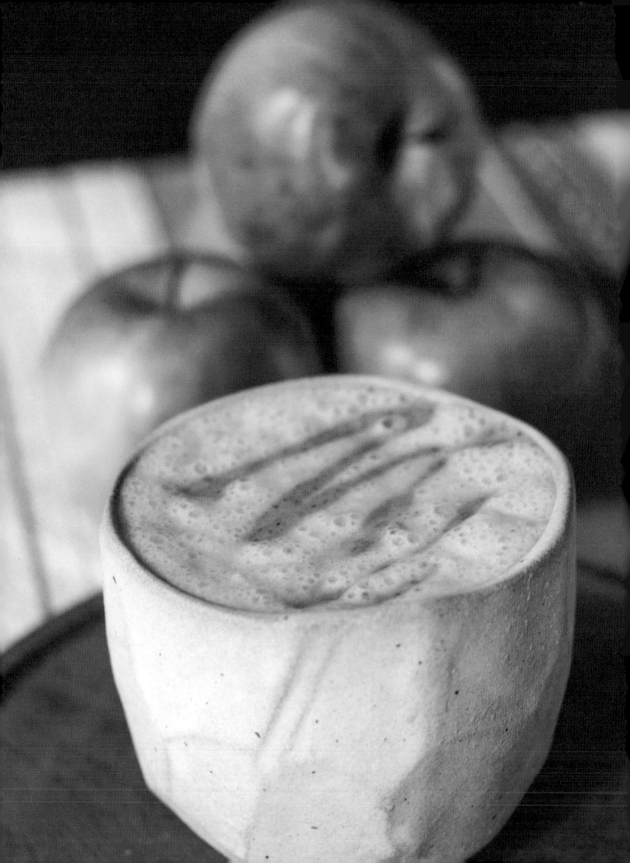

CARAMEL APPLE

Yield: 2 cups

This smoothie is potentially the most satisfying frozen fall beverage. It legitimately tastes like a caramel apple from the fair. Dress up in some layers, make this delicious cup of decadence, and enjoy in the nearest leaf pile!

SMOOTHIE:
- ⅓ cup mylk of choice
- ⅔ cup apple juice
- 1½ frozen bananas
- ½ tsp cinnamon
- ½-inch sliver ginger
- several pieces of ice

DATE CARAMEL:
- 1 tbsp soaked dates or Date Paste (p 25)
- 1 tbsp almond butter
- 1 tbsp coconut oil
- pinch Himalayan salt

Blend all smoothie ingredients together until super smooth. Blend together the Date Caramel ingredients until combined into a caramel texture. Drizzle the date caramel on top of the smoothie and enjoy!

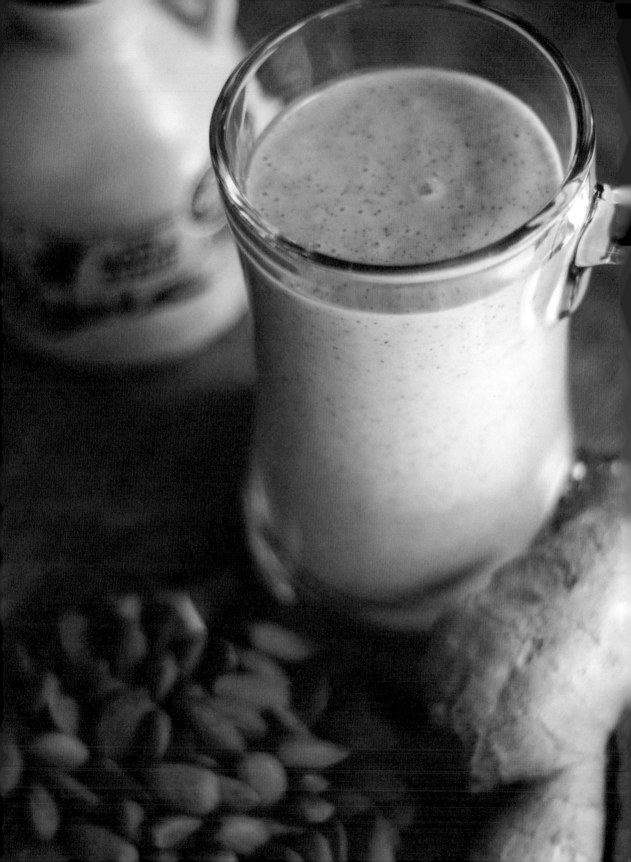

GINGER SNAP

Inspired by a good friend and former Superfresh! server, this is the smoothie version of a ginger snap cookie. We use probiotic ginger ale (a great way to infuse some probiotic goodness) for an extra spicy ginger kick.

½ cup mylk of choice
½ cup Probiotic Ginger Ale (p 183)
1½ frozen bananas
2 tbsp almond butter
1 tbsp ginger juice
1 tsp almond extract
1½ tbsp pure maple syrup

Blend all ingredients together until super smooth. Sip up the spicy, snappy goodness.

TIP: If you don't have the probiotic ginger ale, either sub cold ginger tea or double the mylk and double the ginger juice and it should taste pretty similar.

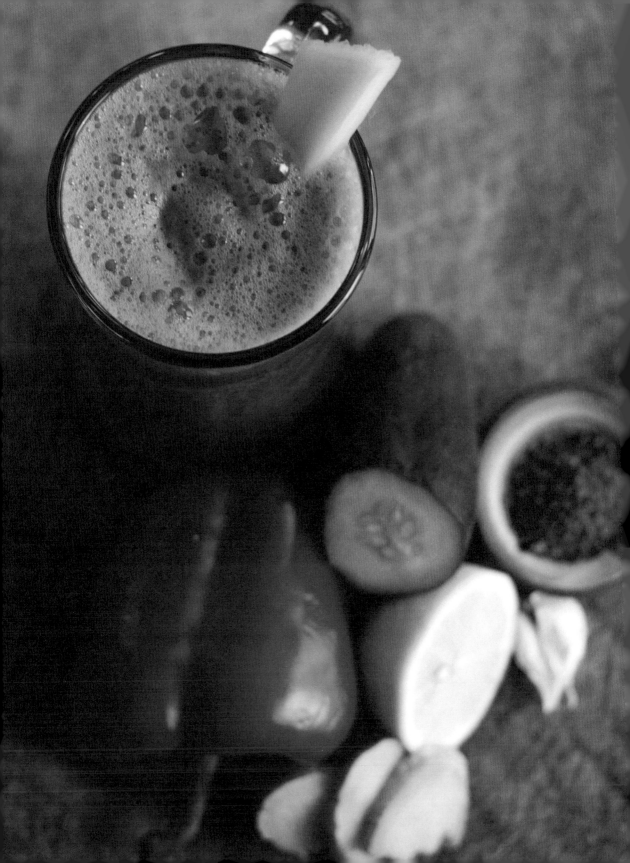

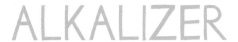
ALKALIZER

Yield: 2 cups

More like a blended raw soup, this savory green smoothie is extremely balancing, and, as its name states, very alkalizing. Enjoy this recipe as a preventative measure to keep your immune system in line, or use it to help your body realign if you're feeling out of whack.

½ cup filtered or spring water
½ cup green juice (Hippocrates Green p 101 or
    Green Goddess p 95 are best)
½ celery stalk
¼ cucumber
2 tbsp lemon juice
½-inch sliver ginger
1 garlic clove
handful of spinach
¼ red pepper
1 tbsp dulse flakes
⅛ tsp cayenne pepper
pinch of sea salt

Blend all ingredients together until smooth. Savor the healthiness and feel your body come back to balance.

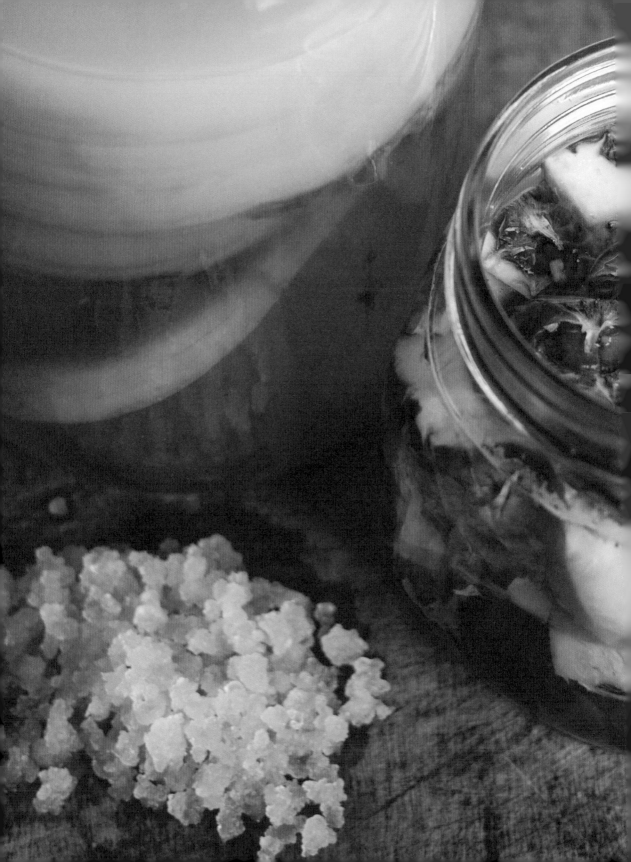

FANCIFUL FERMENTS

Adding fermented foods to your diet increases the vitality of your gut flora (the complex system of microorganisms that live in our digestive tracts), which ripples into boosting your immune system, enhancing brain function, alkalizing your body, and so much more. Traditional Chinese and Ayurvedic medicine (the two oldest medical practices) say that the majority of diseases root from an imbalanced gut. Fermented foods and beverages are an easy and delicious whole food addition to restore and maintain healthy gut flora and, therefore, healthy life!

Fermented drinks have been enjoyed for thousands of years, as they were historically much safer than drinking water.

While the fermentation process of these beverages feeds off sugar that converts into vinegar or alcohol, the fermentation process leaves very minimal amounts of sugar and alcohol in the drinks featured here.

Although you can find many of these drinks at your local health food store or cooperative market, making them at home is extremely easy, far less expensive, and fun! Having glass jars of ferments on your kitchen counter will look beautiful and serve as great conversation starters with company!

The brews take various times depending on the recipe and the environment. Ferments are best kept in a dark space at room temperature while fermenting. Too cool, and they will ferment very slowly; too warm, and they'll ferment super fast (which isn't necessarily a good thing). Refrigerating once complete stops the fermentation process, so your brews won't continue to ferment and turn into vinegar or alcohol.

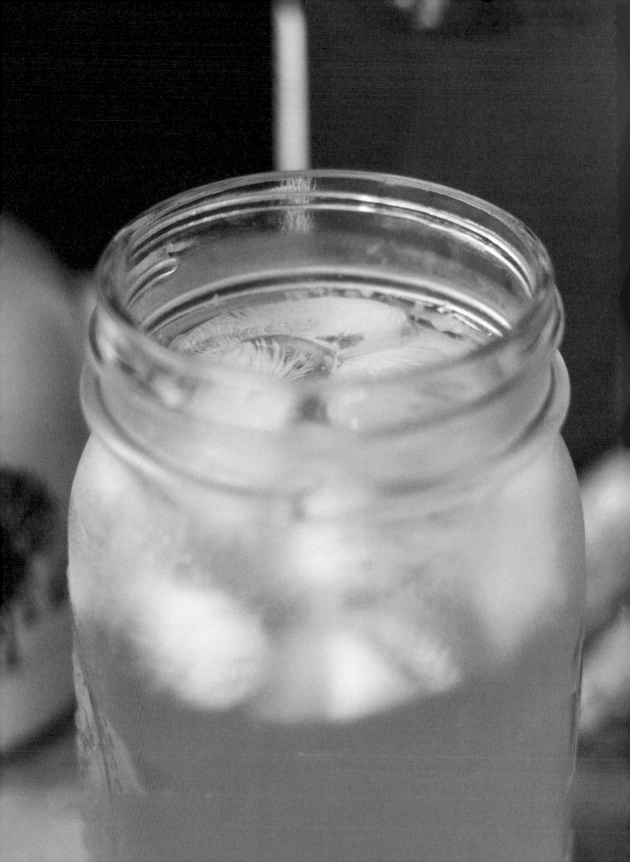

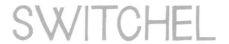

SWITCHEL

Yield: 1 quart

This brew is also known as "haymaker's punch," as it was a staple form of hydration, filled with potassium-rich electrolytes, for farmers during American colonialism, with possible origins in the Caribbean.

Switchel is one of the most simplistic, lightly fermented drinks you can make, as it can take less than 24 hours and has extremely minimal prep.

2 tbsp apple cider vinegar
1 tbsp lemon juice
2-inch fresh ginger root, unpeeled and grated or minced
3 tbsp pure maple syrup or blackstrap molasses
3½ cups filtered water

Put all ingredients into a glass jar. Secure the lid on the jar and shake until well mixed. Let sit in the fridge for 1–2 days and strain before enjoying.

TIP: While you can drink this immediately, it has more flavor and health benefits after a couple days.

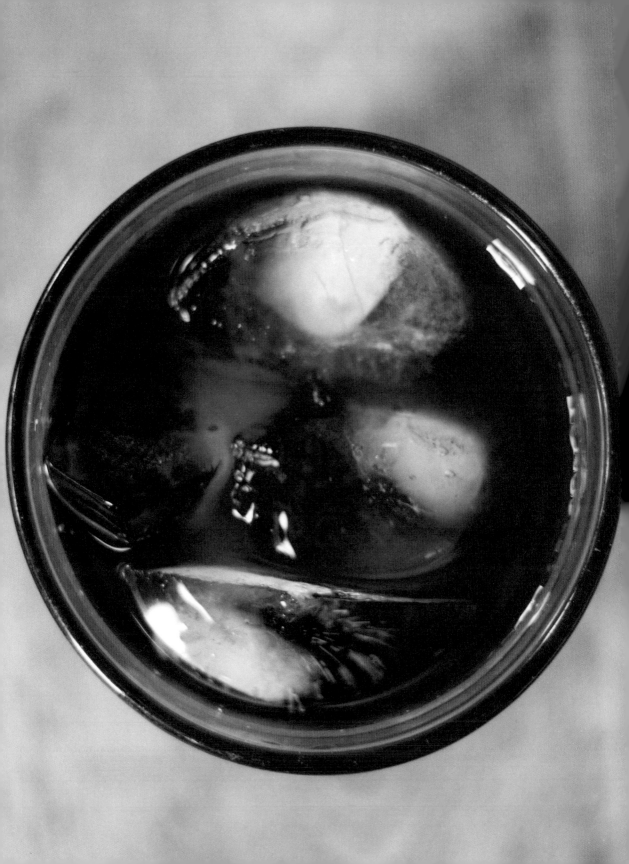

BEET KVASS

Yield: ½ gallon

Beet kvass is a traditional Russian fermented drink that contains beneficial probiotics and enzymes, purifying the blood, boosting energy, treating cancer, and cleansing the liver. This brew has a salty, earthy taste and is usually consumed in smaller doses of 3–4 ounces.

2–4 medium beets, washed and chopped (do not peel)
1 tbsp Himalayan salt
¼ cup sauerkraut juice
filtered water to cover

Add beets, salt, and sauerkraut juice to a half-gallon glass jar. Fill the jar with filtered water, leaving about ½ inch at the top. Cover with a clean rag and secure with a rubber band. Set the jar on the counter, away from the sun, for approximately two days. The temperature of the room will change the rate of fermentation (hotter = faster). Test daily until the desired taste is reached. Strain out the liquid into a clean jar. Seal and refrigerate.

> **TIP:** Combine the Beet Kvass with sparkling water, lime juice, and maple syrup for a delicious spritzer that also makes for an amazing mixer with tequila!

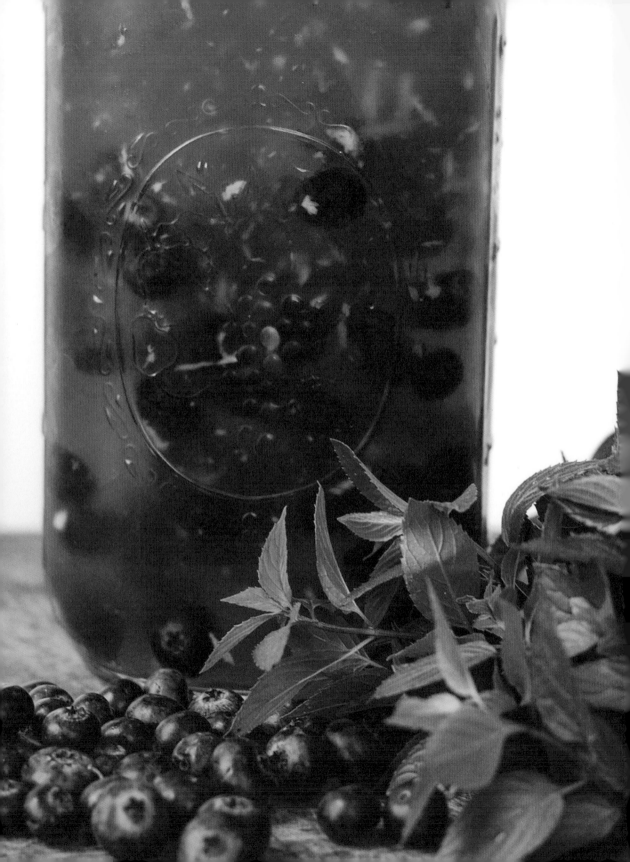

FRUIT KVASS

Yield: 1 quart

Fruit Kvass is one of the quickest fermented beverages to enjoy. The first three ingredients in this recipe are merely one example of many potential combinations. As long as you have fresh fruit, raw honey, and water, and follow the steps, the result will be Fruit Kvass. Feel free to experiment with other fresh fruit, fresh or dried herbs, and spices.

1 cup fresh blueberries, slightly pressed once in jar to break skin
1-inch ginger root, unpeeled and freshly grated
1 sprig fresh peppermint, chopped
1 tbsp raw honey (pasteurized will not work)
3 cups filtered water

Thoroughly clean a 1-quart jar to eliminate potential dirt or bacteria from interfering with the fermentation process. Put the berries, ginger, peppermint, and honey into the jar. Cover with water, leaving 1 inch of air space at the top for pressure.

Tightly secure the lid on the jar and gently shake to mix the ingredients together. Set the jar on the counter, away from the sun, for approximately two days. The temperature of the room will change the rate of fermentation (hotter = faster). Test daily until it reaches the desired taste.

After 24 hours, you should begin to see bubbles from the fermentation process. It is recommended to burp the jar (loosen the lid and tighten it again) daily to prevent the jar from exploding. When the fruit looks cooked and the liquid is bubbly, strain out any solids and bottle your kvass. If you'd like more carbonation, leave it in an airtight jar on the counter for 1–3 days. Once at the desired taste and carbonation, refrigerate and enjoy!

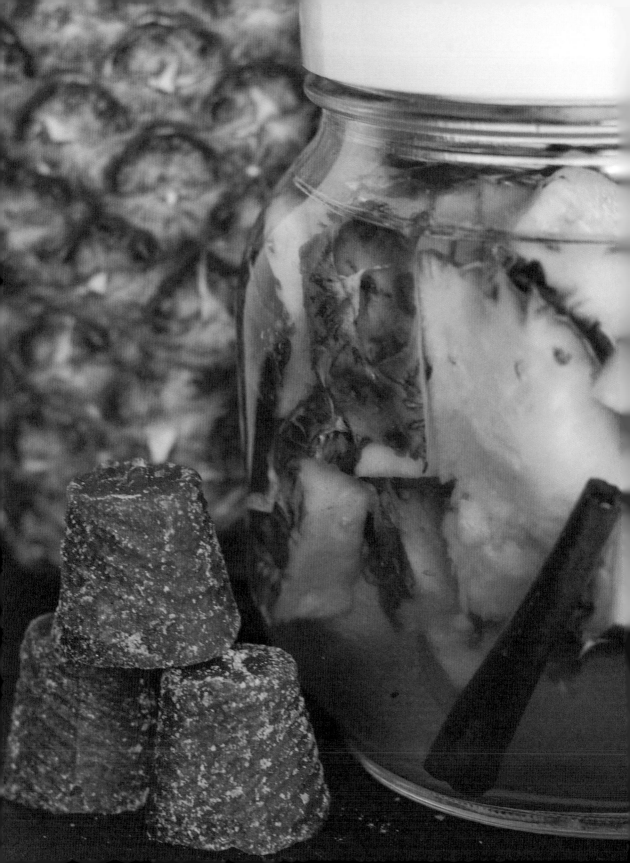

TEPACHE

This Mexican *agua fresca* is a delicious and mild brew with a short fermentation time. It also makes a great mixer!

1 pineapple
1 cup piloncillo or dark brown sugar
1 cinnamon stick
filtered water to cover

Chop the pineapple rind into chunks. Save the fruit to eat, or freeze it for smoothies. Place the rind, piloncillo, and cinnamon stick in a half-gallon glass jar. Cover with water, leaving 1 inch of air space at the top.

Cover the jar with a clean rag and secure with a rubber band. Set the jar on the counter, away from the sun, for approximately two days. The temperature of the room will change the rate of fermentation (hotter = faster). Check at least once a day to ensure the fruit is fully submerged in liquid to prevent mold growth. Test the flavor daily until it reaches the desired taste.

After 24–48 hours, you should begin to see bubbles from the fermentation process. When pineapple rind looks cooked, and the liquid is bubbly, strain out the rind and spices and bottle your tepache. If you'd like more carbonation, leave it in an airtight jar on the counter for 1–3 days. Once at the desired taste and carbonation, refrigerate and enjoy!

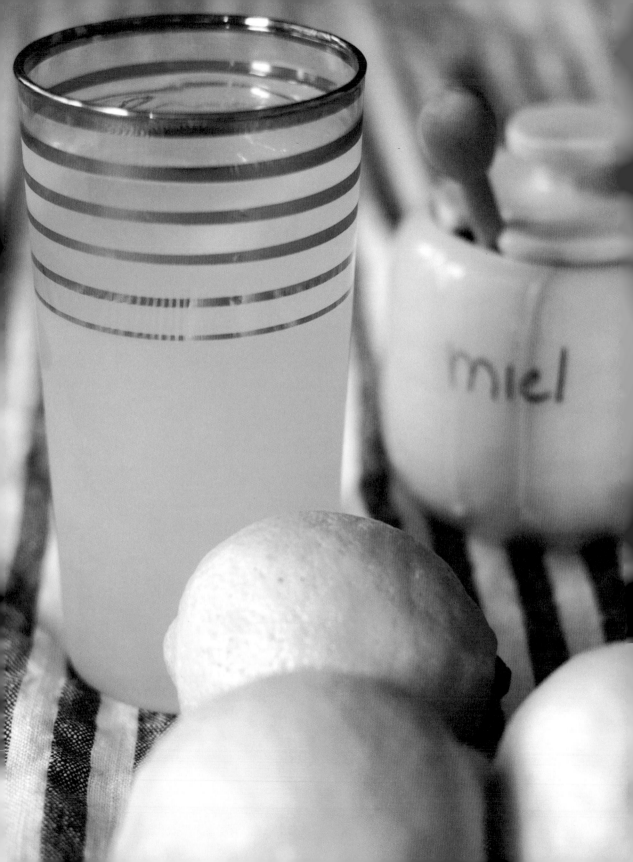

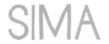

SIMA

Yield: ½ gallon

This Finnish fermented lemonade, originally mead, is traditionally brewed in Finland on May Day to celebrate the beginning of spring.

This is one of the easiest fermented drinks to make at home, and the flavor is very mellow, making it a great introduction to ferments for kids and newcomers.

2 quarts filtered water
1 lemon, thinly sliced
½ cup brown sugar
½ cup raw honey
1⁄16 tsp active dry yeast
2 raisins

Boil 1 quart of water in a medium saucepan. Lower the heat and add the lemon, sugar, and honey. Stir and let cool. Add the remaining quart of water. Once the mixture is lukewarm, add the yeast. Pour into a half-gallon jar and cover with a clean rag or cheesecloth. Let sit at room temperature for about 24 hours. Strain the liquid into another half-gallon jar, add the raisins, cover, and store in a cool place. Once the raisins float to the surface, the brew is ready to drink! Refrigerate in a sealed container.

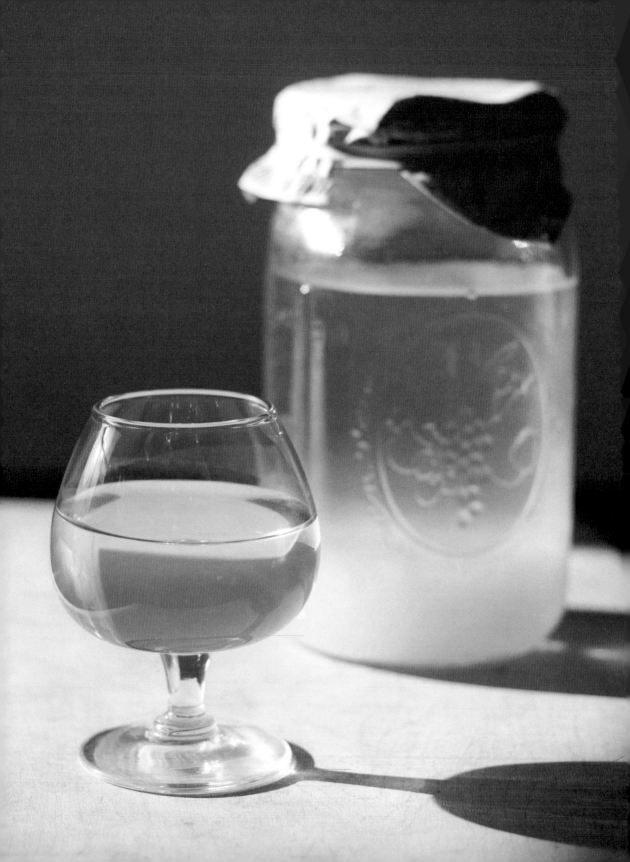

WATER KEFIR

Yield: 1 quart

Water kefir grains are used as a dairy-free alternative to making kefir, a naturally carbonated, lacto-fermented beverage that can be flavored in a variety of ways. The grains are not actually grains, but a combination of bacteria and yeast.

---

6 cups filtered water
1 cup raw cane sugar
1 packet water kefir grains, see Sourcing (p 230)

To make sugar water, heat ½ cup of water in a teakettle or small saucepan. Remove from heat and add ½ cup of sugar, stirring to dissolve. Add 2½ cups of room temperature water.

To activate the grains, transfer the sugar water to a 1-quart glass jar. When the water temperature is between 68 and 85 degrees F, add the kefir grains. Cover the jar with cheesecloth, a coffee filter, or clean rag and secure with a rubber band. Set the jar in a warm spot (between 68 and 85 degrees F) for 3–4 days. Strain the activated kefir grains and gently rinse in lukewarm water, discarding the sugar water.

To make the kefir, prepare a new batch of sugar water using the same steps as above. Put the sugar water into a 1-quart glass jar. When the water temperature is between 68 and 85 degrees F, add the activated kefir grains. Cover the jar with cheesecloth, a coffee filter, or clean rag and secure with a rubber band. Store in a warm spot (between 68 and 85 degrees F) for 24–48 hours. Strain the liquid into a clean glass jar and cover. Refrigerate and enjoy!

> TIP: Make sure to save the grains after each brew to reuse for the next batch! In time the grains will likely multiply, and you can begin to use more sugar water, resulting in a larger yield size.

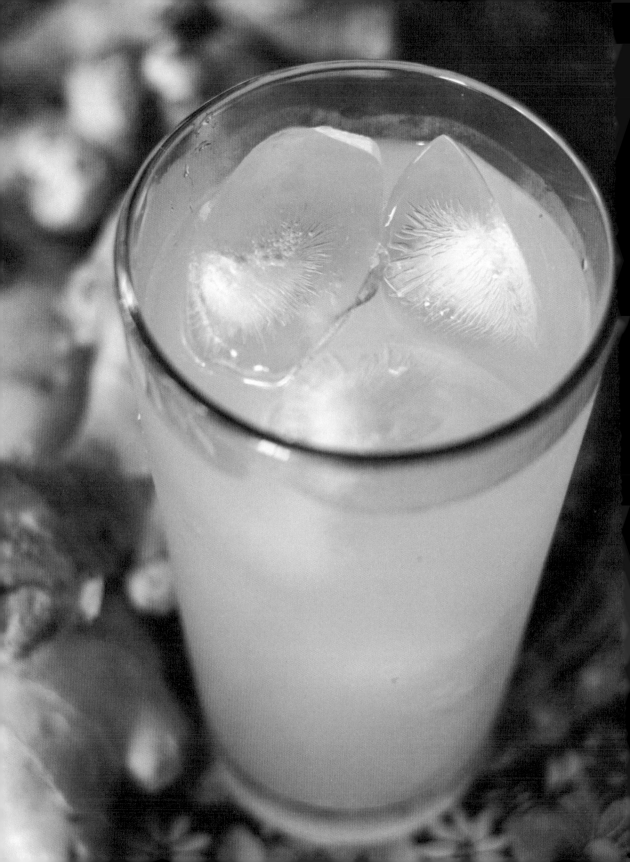

PROBIOTIC GINGER ALE

Ginger ale is my personal favorite soda, but as I no longer drink most store-bought varieties (except the occasional bottle of natural brew), this easy fermented drink is an exciting addition to my staple pantry!

It starts with making the ginger bug, which is a wild fermentation process with a final result that can be used as a base for most natural sodas.

GINGER BUG:
- 1–2 pieces fresh ginger root, grated (do not peel)
- ½ cup raw cane sugar
- 2 cups filtered water

GINGER ALE:
- 7 cups filtered water
- ½ cup freshly grated ginger root or ginger juice pulp (fresh, frozen, or dehydrated)
- ½ cup raw cane sugar
- 1 cup Ginger Bug

To make the Ginger Bug, place 2 tbsp of grated ginger and 2 tbsp sugar into a clean 1-quart glass jar. Add 2 cups of filtered water and stir. Cover with cheesecloth, a coffee filter, or clean rag and secure with a rubber band. Store at room temperature.

Every day for the next 5–8 days, add 1 tbsp grated ginger and 1 tbsp sugar and stir. Once bubbles begin to form, it is ready to use.

To make the Ginger Ale, in a medium saucepan, bring 7 cups of water to a boil. Reduce the heat to low, add the ginger root and steep for 20–30 minutes, until you have a strong ginger tea. Turn off the heat and add ½ cup of sugar. Stir to dissolve. Allow the tea to cool, then strain the liquid into a half-gallon glass jar. Add the ginger bug* and cover with cheesecloth or a clean rag. Secure with a rubber band and let sit at room temperature for 2–3 days. Refrigerate in a sealed container and enjoy!

*Do not add ginger bug until the tea is at room temperature, as the heat will kill the culture.

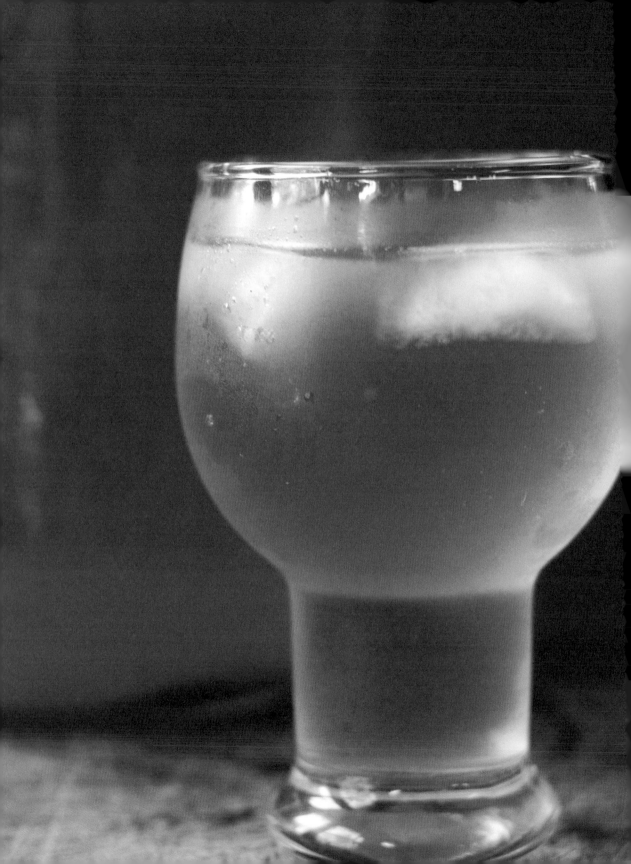

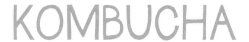

KOMBUCHA

Yield: ½ gallon

This fermented drink, with origins in Russia, has become extremely popular in the health food world over the past decade. It is high in B vitamins and very easy to make at home, so put your wallet away, brew up, and reap the amazing benefits!

7 cups filtered water
1 tbsp loose leaf black tea
½ cup raw cane sugar
1 cup kombucha starter
SCOBY

Thoroughly clean a half-gallon glass jar to eliminate potential dirt or bacteria from interfering with the fermentation process.

Bring the water to a boil in a medium saucepan. Turn off the heat and add the tea. Steep for about 5 minutes. Strain the liquid into jar, add the sugar, and stir until sugar has dissolved. Let cool to room temperature (68–85 degrees F). Add kombucha starter and SCOBY.

Cover the jar with a clean rag or coffee filter and secure with a rubber band. Allow the brew to sit in a cool (68–85 degrees F), dark place for 7–20 days, or to taste.

The warmer the space, the faster the brew time. Through fermentation, the bacteria eat the sugar and turn to vinegar. By day 7, begin tasting the kombucha daily to make sure it doesn't become too vinegary.

TIP: SCOBY is an acronym for symbiotic culture of bacteria and yeast. You can buy kombucha scobies and starter online (see Sourcing, p 230), or find someone who brews (try asking at your local health food store) and will very likely have plenty of extra to go around, as they regenerate rapidly.

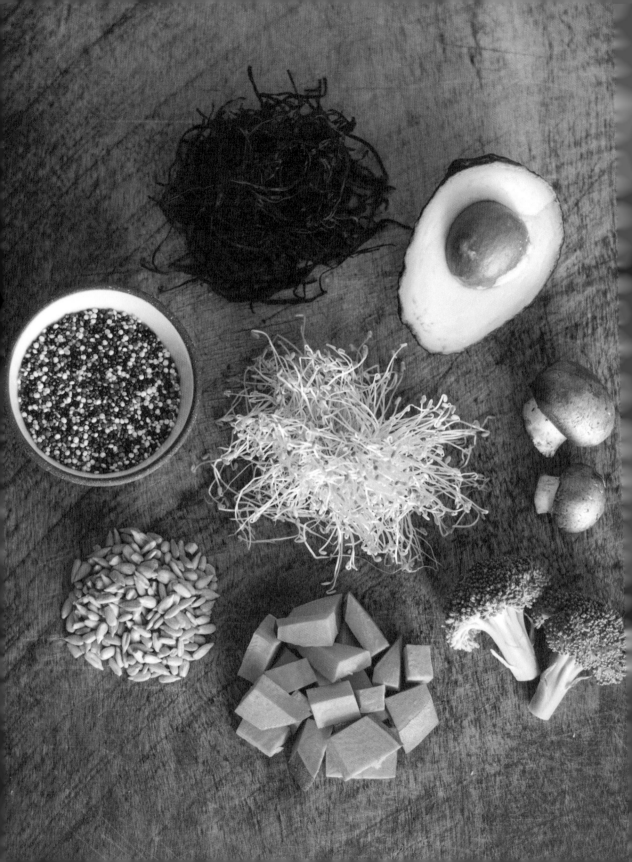

NOURISHING CLEANSES

In this chapter we'll explore my top three go-to cleanses: Raw, Candida / Alkaline, and Ayurvedic. Cleansing is beneficial as it allows our overworked bodies to slow down and recharge with nourishing foods, remove toxins that naturally build up simply by existing, and clean up shop to keep going full steam ahead.

All of these cleanses include food, so you don't have to feel as deprived as you might on a strictly liquid detox, like a juice cleanse or the Master Cleanse (p 29).

They are all also very flexible on their timelines. You can go for one day, a few days, a week, or longer, depending on what your body needs and what your schedule allows.

Technically speaking, the Raw Cleanse and the Alkaline / Candida Cleanse principles can be entirely sustained for the long haul as permanent dietary changes if so desired. Whereas, the Ayurvedic cleanse is recommended for 10–14 days, or as long as needed to get the desired results, with principles and practices that are beneficial when incorporated into daily life.

I usually choose which cleanse I'm going to do based on two key factors: 1) how I'm feeling physically and emotionally; and 2) the season / weather. For instance, the Ayurvedic Cleanse, while wonderful year-round, is perfect in the fall and winter, as it is very warming. The Raw Cleanse is ideal in the spring and summer; my body craves at least some cooked foods in the colder months. If you live in warmer climates, this note is not as pertinent. The Alkaline / Candida Cleanse works any time of year, as it incorporates both raw and cooked foods.

There a few different signals to check in with to decide if it's the right time for you to start a cleanse. The change of seasons is a great time to do a cleanse, as it can already be a difficult time for our bodies to transition with the shifts, and it's a natural time for change. The supportive, gentle, and nurturing nature of cleansing aids us during this change. Another very clear time is when our bodies are calling for extra TLC, or when we are about to embark on a big project that is going to demand a great deal of energy. We are blessed to have vehicles that communicate so clearly with us—the trick is to learn how to listen (an ever-changing daily practice). I can tell it's time to cleanse when I feel a bit sluggish, under the weather, or simply off. This may also be aligned with a more serious health issue that you're working on healing; in this case, I highly recommend working with a health professional (e.g., naturopath, chiropractor, herbalist, and / or holistic doctor) to support and monitor you on your journey.

Finding the right time in the middle of our hectic lives can seem impossible, as no time is really ever ideal. We can find endless excuses with holidays, gatherings, parties, birthdays, celebrations, weddings, busy schedules, etc. But when push comes to shove, our bodies will force us to slow down, usually in the form of becoming sick and restricted to our beds for days (if we're lucky). I had this happen to me just after college. I had known for about a year prior that I really needed to do a Candida Cleanse, as major health issues arose, hindering my daily life. I knew what was wrong (for the most part), I knew what I needed to do, and I kept making excuses, such as I was too busy to cook all of my own food (even though I knew how and loved cooking). After more than a year of this, my health deteriorated so much that doing an intense cleanse was the only option. My two biggest issues were that I was sleeping 14–16 hours a day and still living with major fatigue, and I had constant, extremely painful neck and back pain—and I was only twenty-two! I began seeing a chiropractor three times a week, incorporated occasional acupuncture and craniosacral massage work, had massive amounts of blood work done, followed a strict Candida Cleanse for three months, and implemented a firm supplement regimen with probiotics, B-complex, iron, and vitamin D.

Incorporating healthy lifestyle practices into our daily lives and doing short cleanses once or twice a year can make all the difference in nourishing our bodies so we don't completely hit the wall. In the grand scheme of things, a cleanse is a very brief blip of time in our usually long existence, and it makes the ride much more vibrant!

Recruiting a friend or loved one to join you on this adventure is very beneficial, as you can support each other through the process. This is especially helpful for your first cleanse, as it can be an intense period of time in a difficult, yet beautifully transformational way. At the very least, find someone close to you who is supportive of your decision.

When preparing to begin a cleanse (specifically one longer than 1–3 days), it is important to not jump right into a drastic dietary change, but instead ease your body into it with a few transition days. To help with the transition, begin by cutting out all processed foods and sugars, alcohol, caffeine, animal protein (meat, fish, eggs, dairy), gluten, and soy. The same method of transition can be applied for re-entry back to your daily diet; however, it is highly likely that you will have a newfound perspective on your consumption after a cleanse. As our bodies clear out, heal, and strengthen, and as we learn how to better listen to them, it is rare that we want to add in everything we have cut out purely based on how we feel. For instance, I only have to cut out sugar (minimal raw honey, maple, fruit), alcohol, and caffeine when I cleanse because of where my day-to-day ideal diet has landed. It has taken me more than a decade to find out where I feel my best, and that is always evolving with changes in stress levels, seasons, the environment, etc. My dietary restrictions are a reflection of my body's reactions to the food I consume. While I do eat small amounts of sugar and drink minimal caffeine and alcohol on occasion, I also take breaks when I'm feeling worn out.

While all bodies are different and require diverse needs for optimal health, it is generally agreed upon that we all thrive better by consuming more organic whole foods, mostly plants, and eliminating processed foods and refined sugar.

If possible, when planning your cleanse, try to schedule your first few days on a weekend when you'll have plenty of downtime. Day three is often the hardest one to get through, but I find that once you've hit day four, the power and control shifts, and everything moving forward feels like smooth sailing. Your body will be clearing out a lot of toxins, which can be tiring work and may bring up suppressed / unknown emotions. As a part of the clearing out, our skin often breaks out as our body is pushing out toxins; this is natural and will clear up later into the cleanse. You may likely feel a bit lethargic. Feel free to rest as much as needed; you deserve it! It is also a great time to slow down and reflect. Take time to meditate, journal, practice yoga, schedule a massage or acupuncture session, and really pamper yourself! If you're feeling the need for extra deep elimination, schedule a colonic. This time is all about you rejuvenating yourself to come back refreshed and at your highest potential!

I like to recommend to folks that whenever you get hungry (while cleansing or in daily life) to first drink a glass of water and then see if the feeling is still there. More often than not, the feeling of hunger is actually our body crying out in thirst.

A very interesting side effect of cleansing is how it changes our bodies during the detox and realignment process, and in turn our perspectives on hunger shift. By cleaning up and clearing out we realize that we don't actually need to be eating as much as we do, as long as it is of high quality and nutrient dense. All of a sudden, a little bit goes a very long way in sustaining us!

Sometimes I do as little as clearing out sugar, alcohol, and caffeine from my already gluten-free, soy-free, vegan diet. This simple change can make a massive difference in overall health!

The simultaneous benefit and pitfall of cleaning up your diet and lifestyle is that the cleaner it gets, and the more you are able to truly hear your body's cravings (and moments when it screams for a change), the more sensitive you become to the things you've cut out.

Just remember, no matter what you do, you always have the power to choose again. And any improvement is a step in the right direction. Be gentle with yourself. You are amazing and brave simply because you are open to exploring positive changes.

RAW CLEANSE

This Raw Cleanse is essentially equivalent to a raw food diet. While some raw foodies practice this diet year-round when living in colder climates, many find it is easiest to sustain during warmer months and choose to include some lightly cooked foods in the fall and winter.

It is natural to eat more food when on a raw food diet, as they are not as heavy as their cooked counterparts. Simultaneously, you may sometimes be shocked as to how full you can get on raw foods, especially when incorporating healthy fats like nuts, seeds, and avocados.

Feel free to incorporate any of the drinks in this book into your raw food cleanse. Depending on if you want to completely cut out sugar or not, you can leave the sweetener out of the drinks or swap it for stevia.

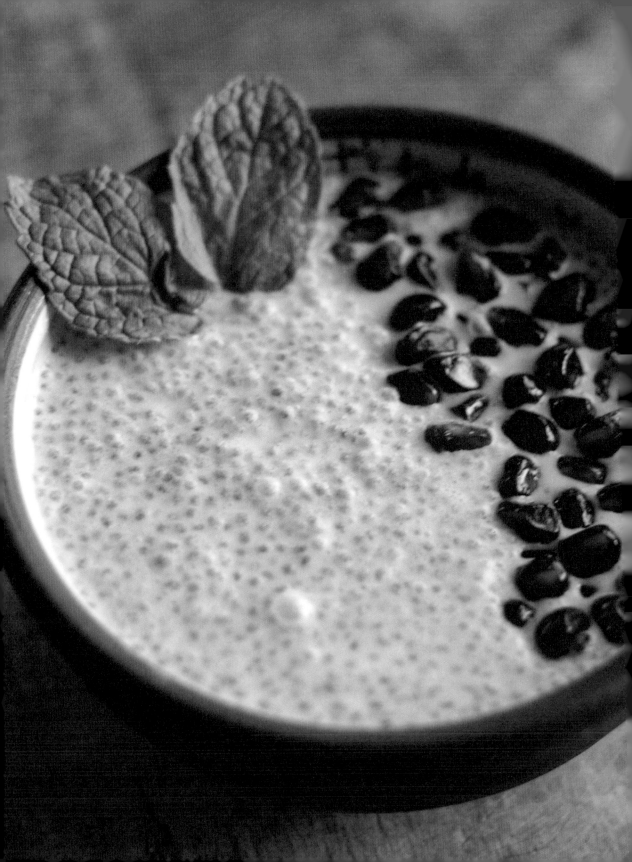

CHIA PUDDING

Yield: 2 servings

This new-age oatmeal is a superfoodie's ode to tapioca pudding. Its creamy goodness is perfect for a filling and energizing breakfast, snack, or dessert.

Feel free to get creative with flavors, superfood add-ons, and dried or fresh fruit toppings.

4 cups mylk of choice
½ cup chia seeds
¼ cup Date Paste (p 25) or liquid sweetener of choice
pinch of Himalayan salt
2 tsp vanilla extract
2 tsp cinnamon
fresh fruit for garnish

Add all ingredients to a small mixing bowl and whisk.* Let sit for at least 20 minutes or overnight before serving.

Whisking when initially adding all ingredients is an essential step, as the chia seeds will clump if not whisked, which is next to impossible to amend after the fact.

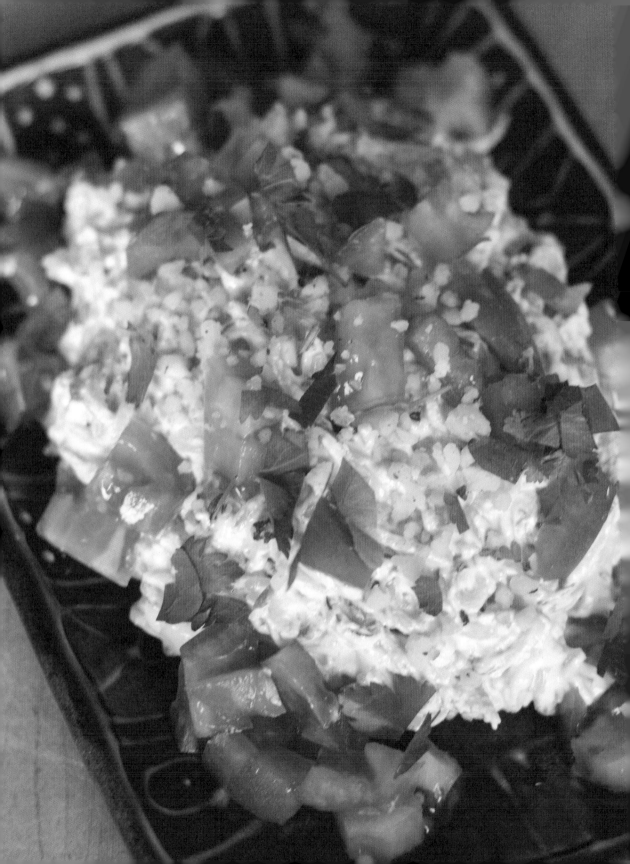

MAC N' CHEEZE

Yield: 2 servings

This is a raw vegan version of a major American childhood classic. Super creamy. Super cheezy. Since the noodles are in a different shape than traditional mac n' cheese, eating it is more reminiscent of spaghetti, however, the flavor is clear. This is perfect for kids!

Feel free to get fancy with this and serve it over a bed of greens (I do that with most of my raw pastas), top it with sautéed mushrooms, avocado, etc. It's such a wonderful base!

MAC N' CHEEZE SAUCE:
- 1 cup raw cashews
- 4 tsp nutritional yeast
- 1½ tsp lemon juice
- ½ tsp Himalayan salt
- ¼ cup filtered water

NOODLES & GARNISH:
- 1 large zucchini, spiralized or grated
- 2 cups kelp noodles
- 2 small carrots, peeled and grated
- 1 tomato, diced
- 4–6 sprigs basil leaves, chopped

Blend all the ingredients for the sauce together until it reaches an extremely smooth consistency. This will take several minutes as it is very thick. Soaking the cashews overnight, and then straining the liquid out before use, makes this process much easier, especially without the help of a high-speed blender.

Toss the sauce into the zucchini, kelp noodles, and carrot until evenly coated. Garnish with tomato and basil. Dig in, and let your memories of grass-stained summers re-emerge.

TIP: If you don't have access to kelp noodles, you can use more zucchini and carrots.

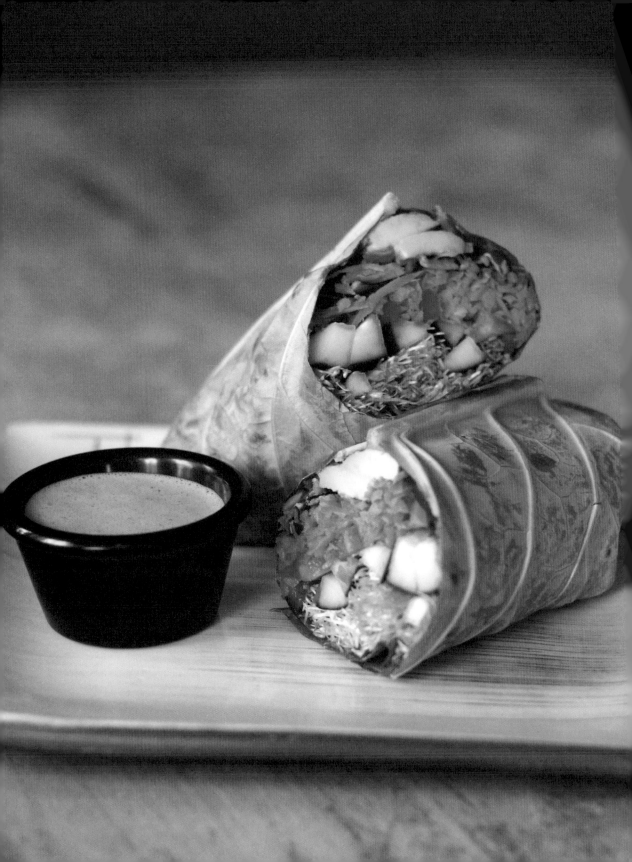

RAINBOW COLLARD SUMMER ROLLS

with Spicy Almond Sauce

Yield: 2 servings

Making wraps in collard leaves is a great way to bypass grain, whether you're on a cleanse or not. These wraps are filled to the brim with so many colors of the rainbow and served with a delicious nutty sauce that's sure to be a crowd pleaser—if you want to share, that is.

2 large collard leaves
½ cup grated carrots
½ cup grated red cabbage
¼ cucumber, julienned
½ red pepper, julienned
½ avocado, sliced
handful of sprouts

SPICY ALMOND SAUCE:
⅓ cup almond butter
⅓ cup coconut aminos
2 tbsp toasted sesame oil
2 tbsp lime juice
2 tbsp pure maple syrup
¼ tsp Himalayan salt
⅛ tsp cayenne pepper (optional)

Add the Spicy Almond Sauce ingredients to a blender and blend until smooth.

Cut out the thicker portion of the collard stem. Place the collard leaves on a cutting board and stack the veggies in the center along the stem line. Fold in the top end of each leaf, followed by the side closest to you. Roll the collard leaves tightly. Cut in half, and serve with sauce.

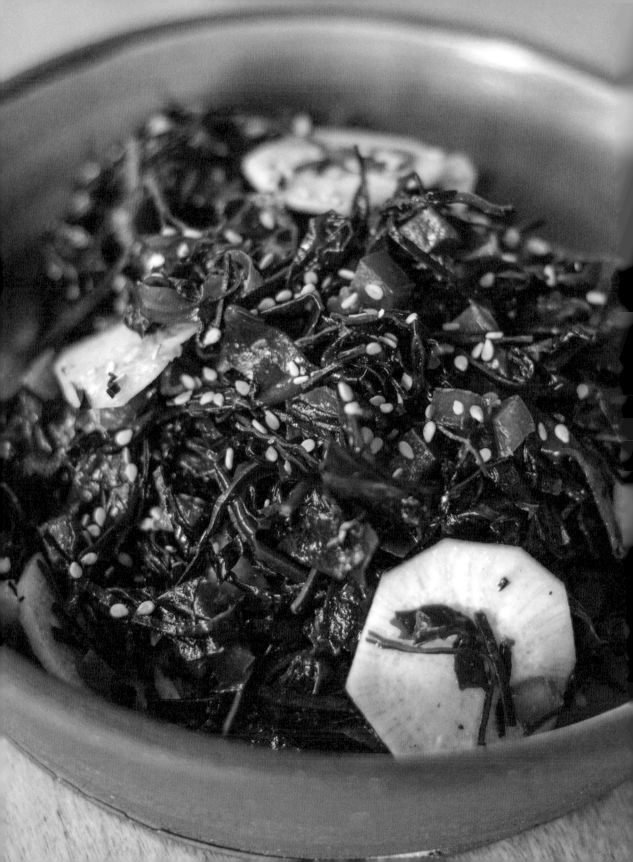

SEAWEED SALAD

Yield: 2 servings

This earthy bowl of scrumptious sea veggies is filled with so much mineral, nutrient-rich goodness that is extremely satisfying on a deep soul level.

2 cup arame
2 cup wakame
¼ red pepper, diced
¾ cup daikon noodles
2 scallions, chopped

SAUCE:
2 tbsp coconut aminos
2 tbsp toasted sesame oil
1 garlic clove
2 tbsp Date Paste (p 25)
¼ tsp Himalayan sea salt
2 tbsp lime juice
½-inch sliver fresh ginger root
pinch of cayenne

Soak the arame and wakame in filtered or spring water for 1 hour. Do not soak more than 2 hours, as they will begin to get mushy, an undesirable texture for this dish. Strain out the liquid.

Add all sauce ingredients to a blender and blend until emulsified.

Add the seaweed, veggies, and sauce to a mixing bowl and toss until well incorporated.

Eat as is, over grain, or serve with greens and enjoy!

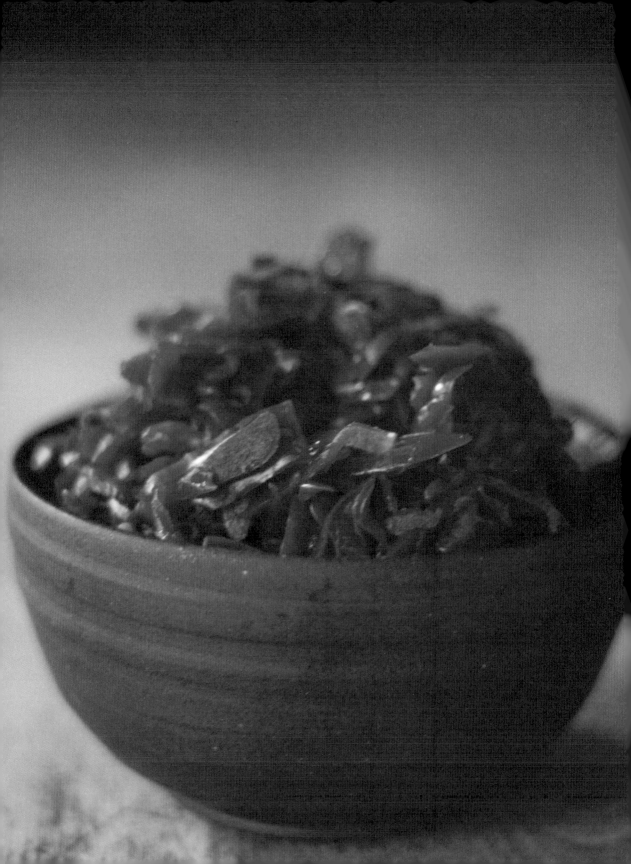

KRAUT

Yield: ½ gallon

Sauerkraut is one of the most well-known, simple fermented foods out there. It also has one of the most basic palettes of all ferments and is a great starting point for newbies.

I enjoy this delicious side dish both plain or as an addition to sandwiches, quesadillas, and more!

1 head cabbage (red or green)
1½ tbsp Himalayan salt

Core cabbage and cut into slices. Massage the cabbage with salt until juicy. You'll be surprised by how much liquid is released! It's truly magical.

Add to a clean half-gallon jar and tamp down until all cabbage is submerged in liquid; if it is not properly covered it will grow mold. You can use a larger cabbage leaf to help keep everything down. Firmly press down a weight (a smaller jar filled with water or a clean rock) on top of the cabbage to keep it submerged. Cover with a clean rag and secure with a rubber band.

Set the jar on the counter for approximately 2 days. The temperature of the room will change the rate of fermentation (hotter = faster). Check daily to make sure the cabbage is properly submerged to prevent mold growth.

Taste test after 2–3 weeks, allow it to ferment until you achieve the desired taste. Then, seal the jar with a lid, refrigerate, and enjoy!

TIP: When you've finished eating the kraut, save the extra liquid in a clean, sealed glass jar. This juice be enjoyed as an immune-boosting shot or as a starter for various fermented recipes, such as Beet Kvass (p 173).

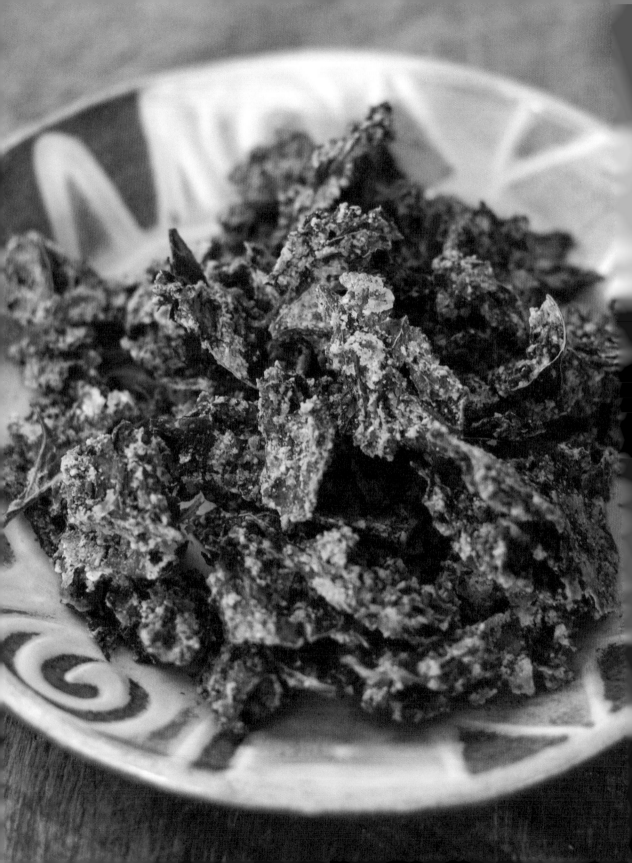

KALE CHIPS

Yield: 2-4 servings

This super trendy snack is extremely easy to make. It can be cooked in an oven at very low heat or dehydrated to preserve its truly raw state and maximum nutritional benefits. Save your hard-earned dough and make this yummy snack at home!

This is a very basic recipe that can be easily adapted. Feel free to experiment with flavors! Add more nutritional yeast for cheezier chips, curry powder for a little Indian flair, or Italian seasoning and sundried tomatoes for pizza flavor; the possibilities are endless!

1 bunch green kale
1 cup soaked sunflower seeds or raw
  cashews
1 tsp nutritional yeast
¼ tsp Himalayan salt

½ tsp cumin powder
1½ tsp lemon juice
¼ cup filtered water
¼ cup coconut aminos
¼ bunch of parsley, chopped

Soak the sunflower seeds for at least 2 hours or cashews overnight in filtered or spring water. Strain and rinse. Add to blender with nutritional yeast, salt, cumin, lemon juice, water, and coconut aminos. Blend until smooth.

Break kale off the stem in chip-size pieces and place in a large bowl. Pour the batter and chopped parsley onto the kale and massage for a few minutes until the kale softens.

Oven preparation: Preheat the oven to the lowest temperature possible. Spread the battered kale onto a cookie sheet and bake for 8–10 minutes.

Dehydrator preparation: Set the dehydrator temperature to 115 degrees F. Spread the battered kale onto dehydrator sheets. Dehydrate overnight, until crisp.

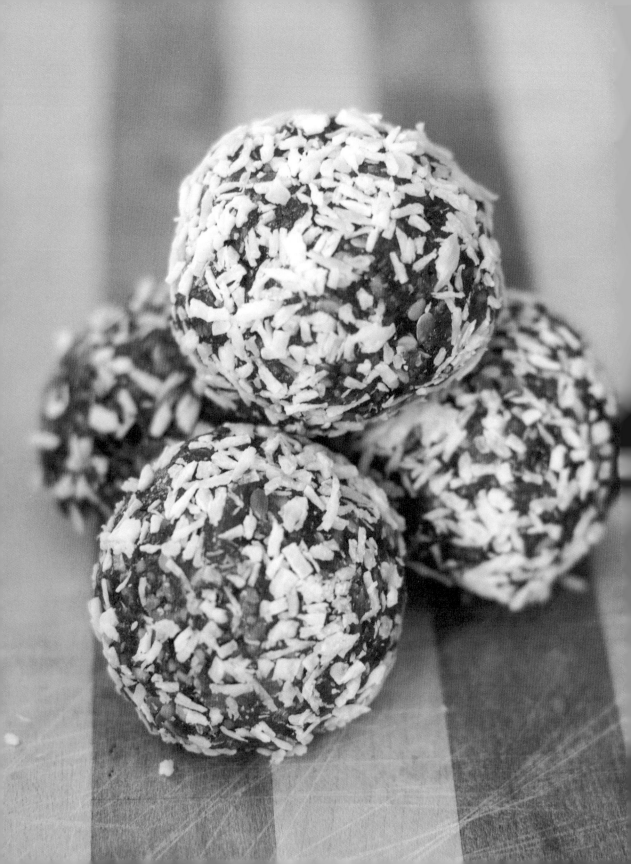

5-SEED SUPERFOOD ENERGY BALLS

Yield: 14 balls

When you're looking for a quick and easy, brain-boosting, protein-rich snack to power you through the remainder of your busy day, look no further than these energy balls. Make a big batch and store them in a sealed container in the fridge or freezer so you can simply grab and go!

1½ cups deglet noor or medjool dates
¼ cup goji berries
2 tbsp cacao nibs (optional)
¼ cup sesame seeds
¼ cup hemp seeds
¼ cup sunflower seeds
¼ cup flax seeds
¼ cup pumpkin seeds
½ tsp Himalayan salt
1 tsp cinnamon
shredded coconut or bee pollen to garnish (optional)

Pit and de-stem the dates.

Add all ingredients except the garnish to a food processor and process until well mixed. The mixture should become a thick batter. Scoop the mixture into a bowl. Roll into eyeball-size balls by hand or with a scoop. Roll in shredded coconut or bee pollen or leave plain.

Feel free to experiment with other toppings, along with other ingredients in the balls themselves. Change it up with added spices or superfoods such as ginger, cardamom, maca, mesquite, or lucuma. This is an easy base recipe that can be transformed into many variations!

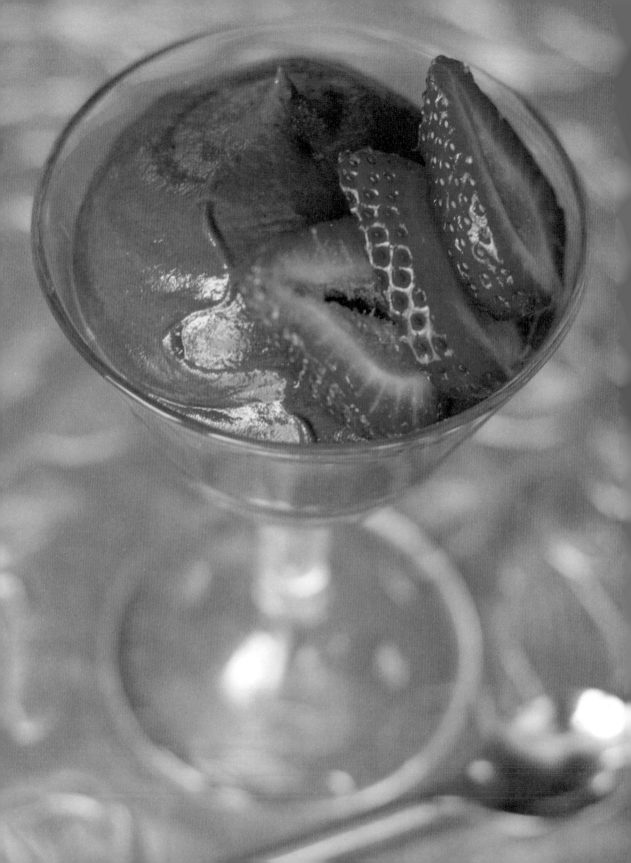

CHOCOLATE AVOCADO MOUSSE

Yield: 2 servings

Every kitchen needs a decadent chocolate mousse recipe. The fact that this happens to be raw and vegan is just a wonderful benefit! Lusciously silky and ridiculously simple to whip up, you will quickly be transported to chocolate pudding heaven!

2 avocados
½ cup raw cacao powder
¼ cup Date Paste (p 25) or liquid sweetener of choice
½ tsp Himalayan salt
1 tsp vanilla extract
1 cup coconut mylk
dash of cinnamon

Add all ingredients to a food processor and process until silky smooth. Refrigerate to set if you'd like a firmer consistency. Top with your favorite superfoods or dried or fresh fruit and enjoy the decadence!

TIP: Feel free to add superfoods like maca, lucuma, holy basil, etc., for a more medicinal punch. See the Superfood Add-On Guide on p 232.

CANDIDA / ALKALINE CLEANSE

The Acid / Alkaline diet is designed to balance the pH of the human body. Much of the Standard American Diet (SAD) is extremely acidic: caffeine, alcohol, sugar, most grains and starches. An acidic diet is the picture-perfect environment for many health problems, including candida overgrowth.

Candida is gut bacteria that's found in all human bodies. Its presence is not an issue when in proper balance, however, when in abundance it is linked to many major health issues. Not only does candida thrive in acidic environments, but it also loves bodies that are stressed, overworked, and not getting enough rest. This is in line with ancient medical knowledge of Ayurveda and Traditional Chinese Medicine, which link all health issues to the gut, or the *hara*.

This is particularly troublesome for most people living in the Western world. I had major issues toward the end of my college career (spurred on by lots of caffeine, alcohol, sugar, loads of stress, excessive work, and little sleep) that led me to an intense three-month candida cleanse and a massive shift in my overall diet and lifestyle that I continue to integrate into my daily life.

While I definitely go in waves of how intensely I practice these habits, overall I tend to:

- Consume minimal sugar; when I do it is usually dates, raw honey, or maple syrup

- Lean toward more alkaline grains (millet, quinoa, buckwheat, amaranth)

- Eat lots of ferments and seaweeds

- Take breaks from caffeine consumption

- Enjoy minimal amounts of alcohol

While on this cleanse, in addition to everything listed in the introduction to this chapter, you need to completely eliminate the following:

- Sesame seeds

- All sugar, including honey, maple, dates, and all fruit except citrus and green apples

- All root vegetables (carrots, beets, etc.), except red potatoes, onions, ginger, and turmeric

- All grains, except millet, buckwheat, amaranth, and quinoa

- Alcohol

- Caffeine

You should add in:

- Probiotics

- Seaweeds

- Ferments

I also tend to use digestive enzymes, especially when cleansing and primarily before consuming grains and legumes.

In addition to the following recipes, feel free to incorporate any of the Raw Cleanse recipes, except the energy balls. For any of the sweets (chia pudding, chocolate mousse, etc.), be sure to use stevia, monk fruit powder, or leave out the sugar all together. These alternatives are much sweeter than their counterparts, so you'll want to use less than you would normally. You can find references on product packaging or online.

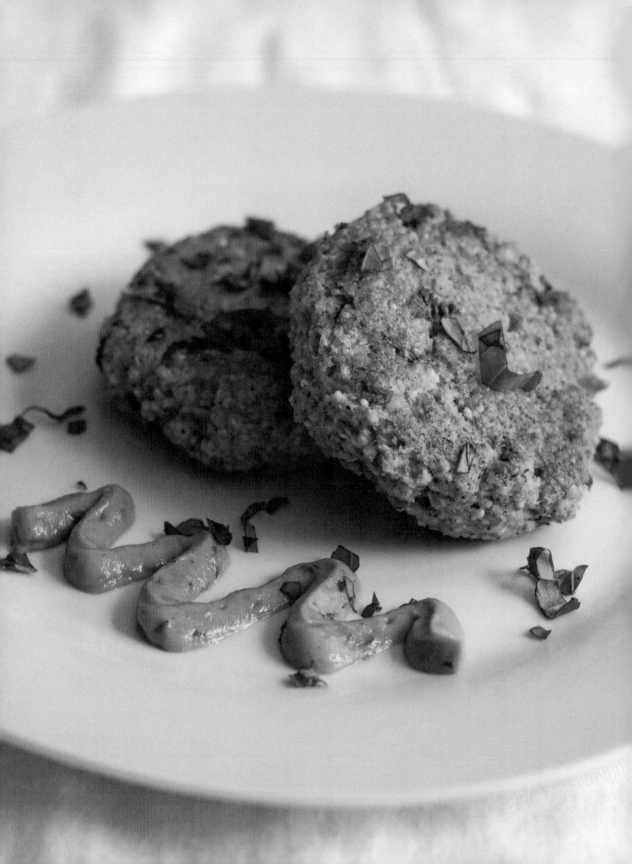

MILLET CROQUETTES
with Avocado Cream

Yield: 17 croquettes

In the beginning of a new cleanse, I usually get super excited and a bit overzealous about all the fancy foods I'm going to make that fit within the detox guidelines. By day three I typically find myself going back to the basics of simple foods that are super easy to whip together, which is my overall outlook on food consumption in my day-to-day home life; I usually save fancy experiments for the Superfresh! kitchen. I made this recipe at the beginning of my first and longest Candida cleanse. They are simple, earthy, grounding, and delicious!

CROQUETTES:
1 cup dried millet
2½ cups filtered water
¾ cup flax meal
¼ bunch of parsley
2 zucchini, roughly chopped
½ onion, diced
3 garlic cloves, minced
2 tsp Himalayan salt
½ tsp ground black pepper
1 tsp cumin powder
olive oil to grease pan

AVOCADO CREAM:
2 avocados
1 cup cashews
1 tbsp lime juice
½ tsp Himalayan salt
2 cups filtered water

Preheat the oven to 400 degrees F.

Add millet and 2 cups of water to a medium saucepan and cook over medium-low heat for 20–30 minutes.

Add ½ cup water, flax meal, parsley, zucchini, onion, garlic, salt, pepper, and cumin to a food processor and pulse until the ingredients are broken down, but still a bit chunky. Add the cooked millet and pulse until incorporated.

Lightly oil a baking sheet with olive oil. Scoop out batter and make small patties (about ¼ cup of batter per patty). Bake for 30 minutes, until golden brown. While the croquettes are baking, put all the ingredients for the avocado cream into a blender and process until smooth. Once the croquettes are done baking, allow them to cool for 5–10 minutes, then serve with the avocado cream.

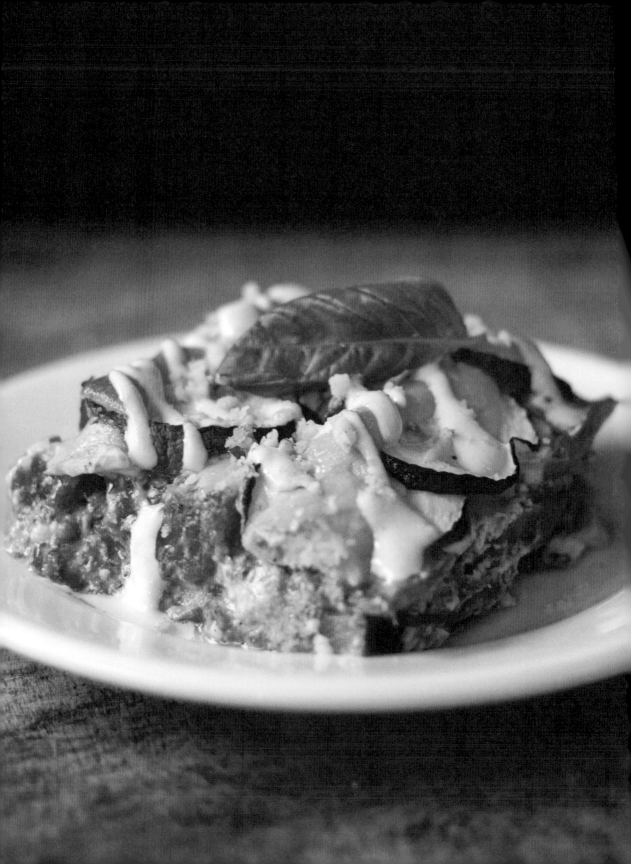

BAKED PALEO LASAGNA

with Cashew Cheeze and Sunflower Seed Pesto

Yield: 4-6 servings

I'm half Italian, and Sunday dinner at my Grandma Erma's house always consisted of spaghetti and meatballs, while lasagna was served far less frequently. But, I simply can't shake lasagna's delicious calling (much more so than spaghetti). This recipe is essentially baked raw lasagna for a warming, melty, classic, nostalgia-inducing dish.

- 1–2 tbsp extra virgin coconut oil or cold-pressed olive oil
- 1 large zucchini, sliced
- 1 medium eggplant, sliced
- 3 medium tomatoes, sliced
- 1 sprig basil and / or parsley, chopped

CASHEW CHEEZE:
- ¾ cup raw cashew pieces
- 1½ tsp lemon juice
- ¼ tsp Himalayan salt
- ⅔ cup filtered water
- ½ tsp nutritional yeast

SUNFLOWER SEED PESTO
- ¾ cup sunflower seeds, soaked
- 2 tbsp lemon juice
- ¼ tsp Himalayan salt
- 4 cups spinach or other greens
- 1 bunch basil

BRAZIL NUT PARM:
- ½ cup Brazil nuts
- ¼ tsp Himalayan salt

Preheat oven to 400 degrees F.

To make the cashew cheeze, put all the ingredients in a blender and process until smooth. It may take a few minutes to break down to a creamy texture. To make the pesto, put all ingredients in a food processor and process until creamy.

To make the Brazil nut parm, add the Brazil nuts and salt to a clean, dry food processor and pulse until it reaches a Parmesan consistency.

Oil an 8-by-8-inch cake pan. Place a layer of zucchini noodles in the pan. Gently spread on half of the pesto. Add a layer of eggplant, followed by a layer of tomato slices. Drizzle with ⅓ cup cashew cheeze. Repeat once. Top with a final layer of zucchini noodles. Drizzle with the remaining cashew cheeze.

Bake for 40 minutes. Check center with a fork to ensure it is tender. Remove from oven and allow it to cool for 5–10 minutes. Serve slices garnished with fresh herbs and Brazil nut parm.

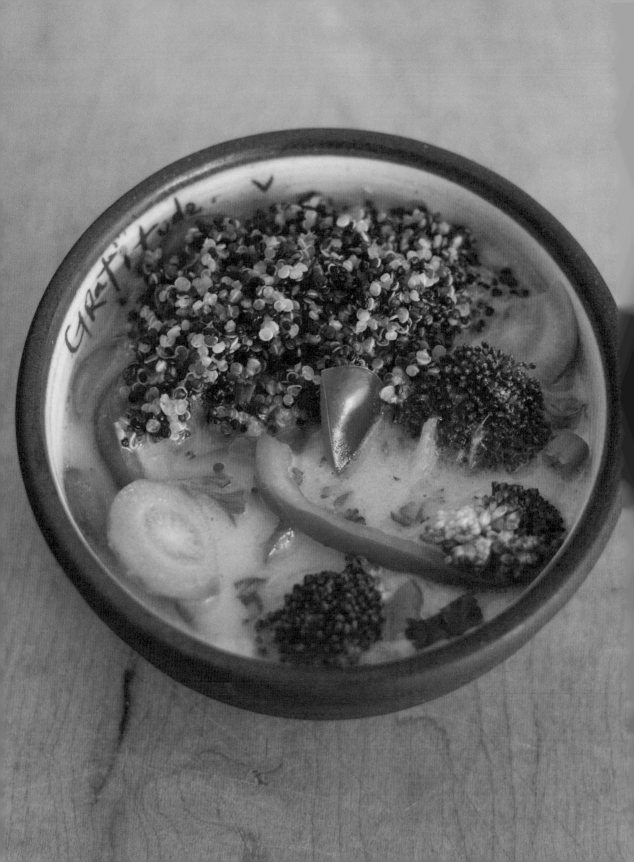

CURRY IN A HURRY

Yield: 4 servings

Curry is one of my favorite go-to dishes. While traditional curries can take many laborious hours of preparation, it's convenient to have at least one good basic curry recipe for those times when you don't have all day to spend in the kitchen. Curries can be extremely simple, and day-to-day home cooking is best when you don't have to make a big fuss or use too many pots—less cleanup is always a plus. This is a great dish to make for dinner parties or potlucks!

2 cups filtered water
1 cup dry quinoa
2–3 tbsp extra virgin coconut oil
½ onion, diced
2 tsp Himalayan salt
1-inch piece fresh ginger root, minced
1 tsp brown mustard seeds
1 tsp cumin seeds
1 medium red potato, chopped

1 medium head broccoli, chopped
1 red pepper, sliced
½ bunch of kale
2 tsp turmeric powder
½ tsp coriander powder
½ tsp ground black pepper
¼ tsp cayenne pepper, optional
2 14-ounce cans of full fat coconut mylk
basil to garnish

In a medium saucepan, bring 2 cups of water to a boil, add quinoa, and cook for about 20 minutes.

Coat a large frying pan or wok with the coconut oil, and sauté the onion and salt over medium-low heat for a few minutes, until golden, stirring occasionally. Add the ginger, mustard seeds, and cumin seeds. Next, add the veggies, turmeric, coriander, and black pepper; if desired, add the cayenne pepper. Cook for a few minutes, then add the coconut mylk. Cook for another 10–15 minutes, or until all the veggies are tender. Serve with quinoa, garnish with basil, and enjoy!

TIP: I always add the hardest veggies first when cooking to give them more time to soften, and then add my greens last. Feel free to vary the veggies in this dish based on what you have on hand and what's in season. This is merely a colorful suggestion.

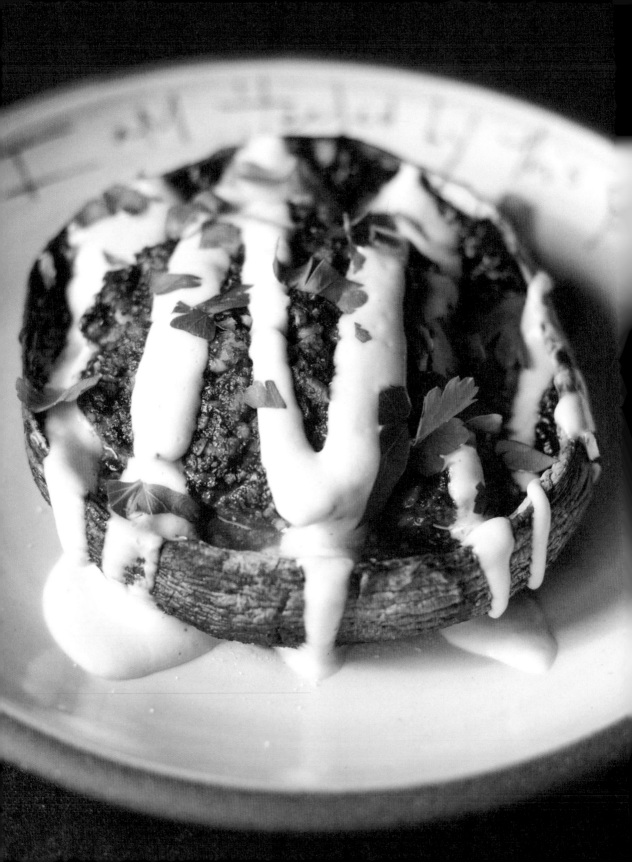

PALEO BAKED & STUFFED PORTABELLAS

Yield: 4 servings

This recipe makes a delicious, filling entrée. Mushrooms are used very frequently in vegan and vegetarian cuisine for a meaty substitute. Filled with a mixture of protein-rich super seeds, delicious veggies, and aromatic herbs, this may easily become a new favorite!

---

4 portabella mushrooms
½ cup pumpkin seeds
½ cup sunflower seeds
¼ medium yellow onion, chopped
1 tsp Himalayan salt
½ tsp black pepper

1 medium zucchini, chopped
2 tbsp fresh or dried oregano
¼ bunch parsley
drizzle Cashew Cheeze (p 213), optional
3 tbsp Brazil Nut Parm (p 213), to garnish
fresh herbs, to garnish

Preheat the oven to 400 degrees F.

Carefully dig out the center of the portabella mushrooms, including the stem, forming a cup for the stuffing. Save the excess mushroom to add to the filling.

Add the pumpkin seeds, sunflower seeds, onion, salt, pepper, zucchini, oregano, parsley, and extra mushroom to a food processor and process until broken down. Don't let it process too long or it will become a smooth paté; this dish is best when the mixture still contains small chunks.

Place the mushrooms on a baking sheet lined with parchment paper. Place heaping scoops of the filling into the portabellas and bake for approximately 25 minutes. Remove from the oven and allow to cool for a few minutes. Drizzle with cashew cheeze and garnish with Brazil nut parm and fresh herbs.

TIP: You can make this fully raw by placing it in a dehydrator at 115 degrees F for 3 hours.

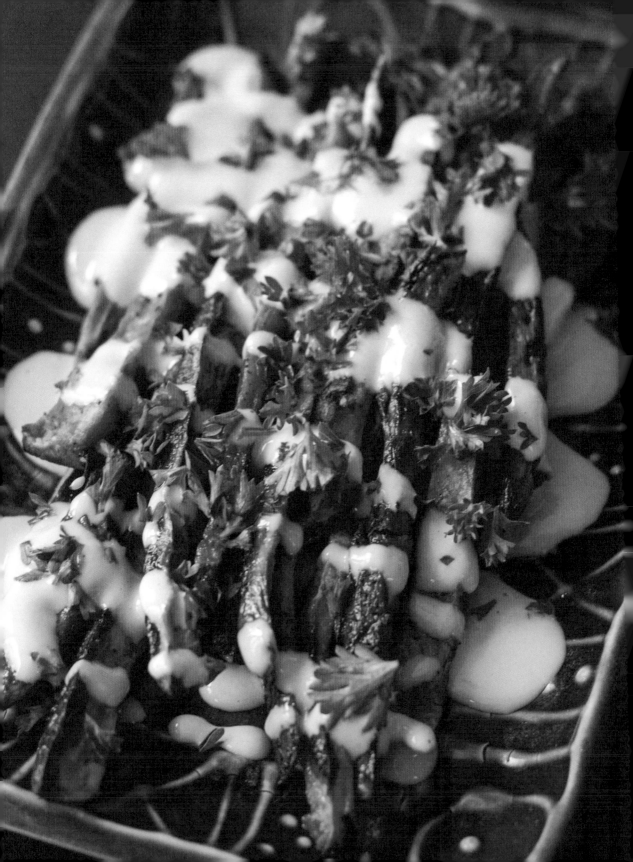

SWEET POTATO FRIES
with Lemon Garlic Tahini
Yield: 1-2 servings

The most simplistic and insanely delicious snack ever; this is easily on my top favorite snacks of all time list! While sweet potatoes aren't technically on the alkaline diet, they are extremely nourishing, easy to digest, and fine in moderation unless you're going through a major health issue, in which case I'd avoid them.

2 large sweet potatoes
¼ cup cold-pressed olive oil
½ tsp Himalayan salt
¼ bunch parsley, chopped

LEMON GARLIC TAHINI:
2 tbsp lemon juice
2 garlic cloves
¼ cup sesame tahini
¼ cup filtered water

Preheat the oven to 450 degrees F. Wash the sweet potatoes and hand cut them. Toss the potatoes with olive oil and salt. Place the fries on a cookie sheet and bake until golden brown, approximately 20 minutes, tossing occasionally.

Put the lemon juice, cloves, sesame tahini, and water into a blender and blend until smooth.

When fries are done, plate and drizzle them with lots of dressing, then garnish with parsley.

Let your taste buds be blown!

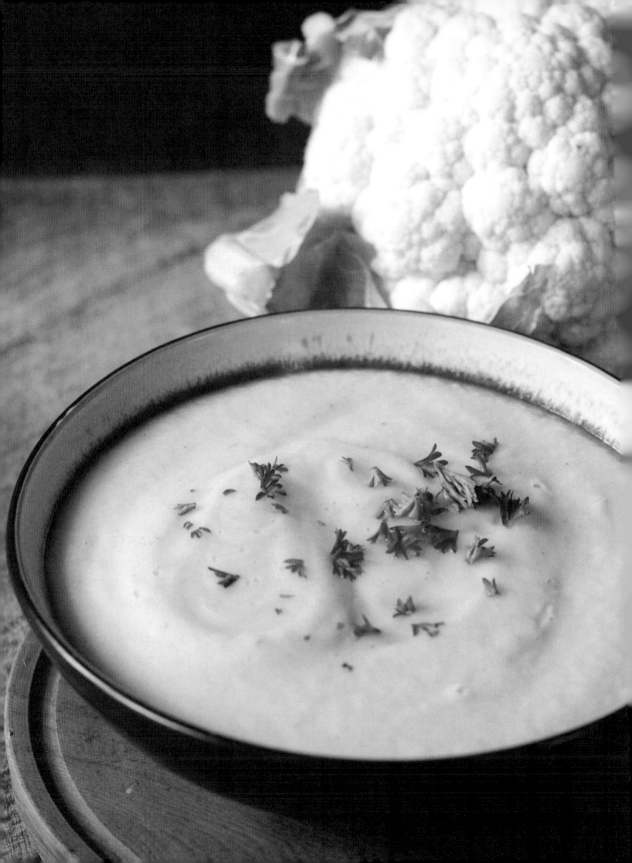

CREAM OF CAULIFLOWER SOUP

Yield: 4 cups

Silky, creamy, perfect for a cool or rainy day. I have an addiction—dipping panini sandwiches into creamy soups—and this soup is perfect for that!

3 tbsp coconut oil
½ medium yellow onion, diced
4 garlic cloves, minced
2 celery stalks, diced
1½ tsp Himalayan salt
1 head cauliflower
1 cup vegetable stock or filtered water
2 cups coconut mylk
½ tsp black pepper

Put the oil in a medium saucepan and sauté the onion, garlic, and celery with the Himalayan salt over medium-low heat for a few minutes, until golden, stirring occasionally. Add the cauliflower and stock or water and allow it to cook down for about 5 minutes. Add the coconut mylk and black pepper and cook until the cauliflower is very soft.

Carefully pour the mixture into a blender and purée until silky smooth. Enjoy!

AYURVEDIC CLEANSE

This cleanse is inspired by a few core Ayurvedic practices. While the other cleanses in this book are more flexible, allowing you to add in other recipes based on the core principles, this cleanse is more specific and you'll want to stick to the basics for the full effect.

Beyond water, the two drinks I include for this cleanse are Golden Mylk (p 59) and Balanced Belly tea (p 15), best consumed after a meal or on their own. The only food consumed is Kitchari (p 225). This permits your digestive system to do very minimal work, allowing it to replenish, strengthen, and stay nourished.

In addition to the diet, I've included self-care practices: dry brushing, Epsom salt baths, tongue scraping, and self-massage. These are wonderful tools that can be incorporated into the other cleanses or your daily lifestyle.

DRY BRUSHING with a special brush (see Equipment p 226) increases circulation, improves lymphatic drainage, and enhances the skin. Brush toward the heart center, beginning with your feet and legs, moving to your stomach and back, followed by your arms. This is best practiced before taking a shower to wash off the dead dry skin and complete the clearing process.

EPSOM SALT BATHS pull out toxins, replenish magnesium, and relieve inflammation and muscle pain. For the full effect, it is best to stay in for 20 minutes. Feel free to add essential oils. Epsom salt baths are best enjoyed at the end of the day before sleep, as you will likely be very tired after the bath. Be sure to drink plenty of water afterwards to replenish your body.

TONGUE SCRAPING removes bacteria, toxins, and dead cells. Its benefits include reducing bad breath, boosting immunity, enhancing digestion, improving sense of taste, and promoting oral health. Stick out your tongue, place the tongue scraper as far back on your tongue as possible, then gently scrape tongue with one long stroke. Rinse off the scraper and repeat 5–10 times.

SELF-MASSAGE, or *Abhyanga*, is a loving practice using warm oil (sesame, coconut, sunflower, almond, or safflower, depending on your dosha) to restore the doshas and promote well-being. Before a bath or shower, gift yourself 15–20 minutes of self-massage, beginning with the crown of your head, followed by your face, limbs (moving toward your heart), abdomen, chest, and feet.

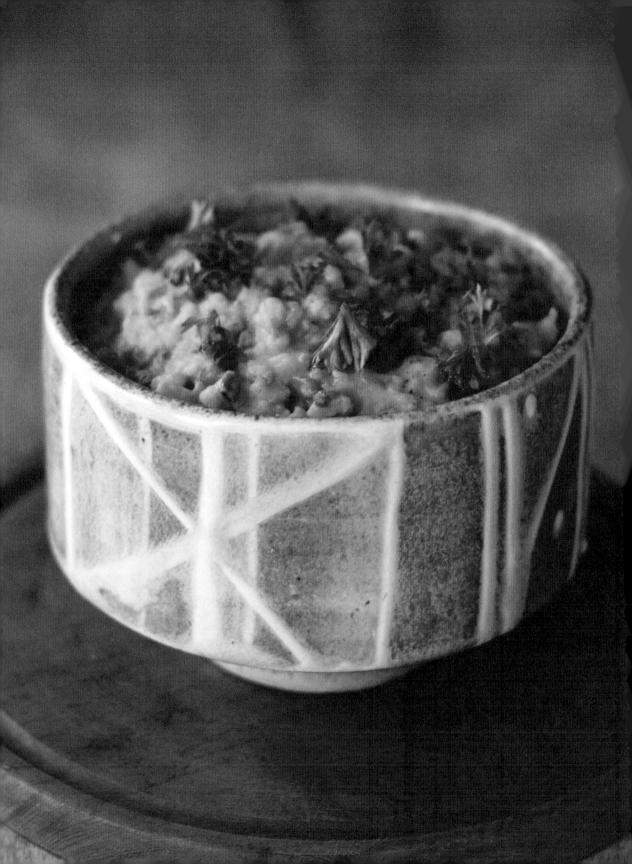

KITCHARI

Yield: 4 servings

This magically grounding one-pot wonder is a nourishing Ayurvedic dish traditionally used as a part of the Panchakarma cleansing process; a ten-day (or longer) detox that is practiced seasonally for prevention and as needed to cure illness.

Kitchari is a mixture of rice and lentils, usually split mung dal. You can add traditional Ayurvedic spices, such as mustard seed, cumin, turmeric, and coriander, as well as veggies, which may vary based on your dosha. Typically made with ghee (clarified butter), I swap for coconut oil in this recipe to keep it dairy-free while still adding many healing benefits, and add coconut mylk for additional creaminess.

This dish is easy to digest while simultaneously improving digestion and balancing the doshas. This is a wonderfully safe cleanse to use year-round and is great during colder winter months.

6 tbsp extra virgin coconut oil
2 tsp mustard seeds
2 tbsp cumin powder
2-inch ginger root, minced
2 tbsp Himalayan salt
2 tsp ground black pepper
2 zucchini, sliced into half moons
2 carrots, sliced into half moons

2 cups dried brown rice
2 cups dried mung beans
2 tbsp turmeric powder
2 tsp coriander powder
10 cups filtered water
3 cups full-fat coconut mylk
½ cup nettle (optional)

Add the coconut oil to a medium saucepan over low heat. Add mustard seeds, cumin, ginger, salt, black pepper, zucchini, and carrots. Stir. After a few minutes, add the rice, mung beans, turmeric, coriander, and water. Cover and let cook for approximately 30 minutes.

Once brown rice and mung beans are fully cooked, add the coconut mylk and nettle, if desired. Stir and cover for a few minutes, until it reaches a creamy consitency.

EQUIPMENT

JUICER: There are two kinds of juicers available: centrifugal and masticating. Centrifugal are generally cheaper than masticating. When I did my first juice cleanse, I bought a $30 centrifugal juicer from a big box store. While I don't recommend that, it's better than not juicing at all. However, you will use much more produce (in turn spending more money), and get less of a nutritional bang with a low-quality juicer.

Centrifugal juicers are designed to press produce down through a mesh basket. They work best with soft or hard produce, while they struggle with leafy greens. There is concern that this style juices at a higher heat and that it creates higher oxidation (i.e., breaking down enzymes for easier assimilation), which is a good thing when done more gently. Because of their structure, centrifugal juicers are often loud.

Masticating juicers (also known as cold-pressed) are generally more expensive up front, but are able to do a great deal more in the long run, saving money by getting the most out of your produce and keeping nutrients more intact, which in turn keeps the juice fresh for longer. These are wonderful for juicing leafy greens and wheatgrass, and are usually also able to grind coffee, make sorbets from frozen fruit, process nut butters, make pasta, and more! Masticating juicers, in general, are less noisy.

Things I look for in a juicer:

- Cleanup ease and time (because you want to actually use it!)

- Versatility

- Longevity of final product (while it's best to drink up immediately for optimal nutritional benefits, some juicers keep juice longer than others—when refrigerated, of course)

- Getting the most out of my produce (watch videos of different juicers and you'll notice that they produce varying amounts of juice)

- Size (too bulky makes it hard to fit on the counter, but too small and you'll be cutting your produce forever trying to make it fit)

- Noise level

- Warranty

My personal favorite is the Omega 8006; I've had mine for about seven years, and it still works like a champ! I've had a couple parts break after extreme use, and the warranty covered it fully, easily, and I got my replacement within seven business days! I also have eight years left on my warranty! Although I dream of someday owning a Norwalk, I doubt I'd ever get rid of my Omega as it's so easy for daily use.

Beginner: Breville JE98XL Juice Fountain Plus (centrifugal, $145)

Intermediate: Breville 800JEXL (centrifugal, $300)

Advanced: Omega 8004 (masticating, $260)
Omega 8006 (masticating, $300)
Green Star GS-1000 (masticating, $450)
Champion G5-NG-853S (masticating, $265)

Super Advanced: Norwalk Model 290 ($2,595)

Pro: This juicer is a very expensive, beautiful machine designed to get the most goodness out of your produce with a very gentle process. It is used by Gerson Therapy Institute for extremely high-quality health practices and is the best of the best if you're looking for premier health results, especially if you're suffering from a major illness, such as cancer or multiple sclerosis.

Con: There are multiple steps, which make the juicing process take longer. Cleanup is much more intricate.

MANUAL WHEATGRASS JUICER: Save electricity and money—try out a manual wheatgrass juicer. Wheatgrass can only be juiced through a masticating juicer. There are high-end commercial electric wheatgrass juicers, but they cost a fortune and don't make sense for home use.

Beginner: Weston Manual Wheatgrass Juicer 36-3701W ($30.99)
Miracle MJ445 Wheatgrass Juicer ($130)

BLENDER: While juicers extract the liquid from whole foods, separating the pulp, blenders keep everything. When I was just starting out I had the blender that was handed down to me from my parents. I eventually swapped it out for a similar thrift store find when it died and didn't get a high-speed blender until I opened my café. Even though they are quite an investment, when you are finally able to make the plunge and benefit from the magic a blender like the Vitamix or Blendtec can create, your world will never be the same, and the creative possibilities in your kitchen will be boundless!

Intermediate: Nutribullet High-Speed ($80)
       Ninja NJ600 ($100)

Advanced: Vitamix Refurbished ($329)
       Vitamix 5200 ($449)
       Blendtec ($400)

FOOD PROCESSOR: Some of the recipes in this cookbook use this standard kitchen appliance—it's one that I and definitely Superfresh! could never live without. Food processors allow you to roughly chop ingredients for recipes like salsa or blend further (but not too much) for spreads like hummus and pesto. I had a very small home food processor for years and eventually upgraded to a larger size so I didn't have to struggle so much with it overflowing. When I discovered that I could also slice or grate veggies with attachment blades, my life was officially changed, and my hands were saved from hand grating! I find this is especially helpful when grating carrots, beets, zucchini, or cabbage, or for slicing large amounts of onion or veggies for fermenting.

SPIRALIZER: This is such a fun, affordable (about $30) kitchen toy that is great for kids. Do be a bit careful though, the blades are quite sharp! I prefer the countertop versions over handheld, as I find they are much easier when spiralizing hard veggies or even a large quantity of zucchini noodles.

NUT MILK BAG: While I have been known to not strain my mylk at home on occasion, it is ideal to use a bag (especially if you don't have a high-speed blender) for a more desirable consistency.

DRY BRUSH: This is an affordable ($6–$20) home spa tool that can be found online or at your local health food store. They are usually made with vegetable fiber bristles and a bamboo handle. Yerba Prima makes one with a long, removable handle.

TONGUE SCRAPER: There are several different styles of plastic or stainless steel tongue scrapers. I prefer stainless steel. Find one online or at your local health food store for under $10.

WATER FILTER: There are so many water filters on the market that finding the best one within your price range can be a daunting task. For the most part, whatever water filter you get is better than no filter at all. The easiest setup would be a pitcher, slightly more advanced would be a faucet attachment, and the next step would be an under-sink system. There are other varieties, such as countertop, reverse osmosis softeners, and whole house systems. Check out the Environmental Working Group's "Updated Water Filter Buying Guide" online for a more detailed list tailored to fit your needs. *Note: the prices below do not reflect necessary filter replacements.*

Pitchers:	Pur 2-Stage ($12.99 - $30) Brita LP Water Filtration Pitcher ($18.44 - $29.99)
Faucet Attachment:	Brita LP Faucet Filtration System ($38.58) Pur Classic Faucet Mount ($16.99 - $62.45)
Under-Sink:	Aquasana 3-Stage Claryum Water Filter System ($199.99)

COLD BREW COFFEE BREWER: There are many varieties on the market. My favorite, and the brand we use at the café, is the Toddy Cold Brew System. We use the commercial model, but I recommend the home model, which is available online for $39.99.

SOURCING

You can find the ingredients listed in this book at your local health food store, cooperative market, farmers' market, farm stand, or online.

CLEAN, LOCAL, SEASONAL FOODS

I highly recommend eating non-GMO, organic foods, especially when it comes to produce. Some produce, usually those with tougher skins and outer layers (like avocados and onions), are safer to buy conventionally than more permeable fruit like strawberries, apples, and celery. Check out the Environmental Working Group (EWG) "Dirty Dozen" food list for more specifics. Removing these pesticides from your diet and body will increase your health and aid in your overall well-being.

Shopping locally and in season is a fun and healthy way to socialize and stay engaged in your community, as well as support your local economy. Eating locally and in season also connects us with the seasons, which helps to reset your internal clock, regulate your digestive system, and provide a generally balanced feeling.

Going to the farmers' market in town or farm stand down the road will likely also introduce you to new foods that you've never seen or tried before! Farmers love sharing their favorite recipes for more unusual crops, so make sure to ask. Many CSA (community supported agriculture) shares also offer this perk for their shareholders, sending out emails with fun recipe ideas.

It can take many years, big piles of paperwork, and a decent chunk of change to become certified organic. Ask your farmer about their growing practices—many practice organic principles, but are unable to afford the certification.

WATER

Water is the backbone of everything you will find in this cookbook, whether or not the recipe actually calls for water or not. You'll notice I recommend using filtered water. If you have access to clean spring water, that is even better, but for the majority who do not, finding a good filter is definitely worth your while. If you're travelling or live in the country check out the website FindASpring.com to find the closest spring.

This major resource necessary for life on earth is highly contended in the world today, between water wars, big oil, big business, and old faulty systems, just to name a few. While this could be an entire book on its own, I will leave you with the recommendation to purchase a water filter (see Equipment, p 226, for more information) and take control as best you can. This is your health after all, and why add all the superfoods if you're going to wash it down with contamination. While this subject is very daunting, my best piece of advice in regards to your home is to do what you can for yourself and your loved ones.

Here Are Some of My Favorite Sources:

Ceremonial Cacao: Heartblood Cacao, www.heartbloodcacao.com

Fermentation Starters and Tools: Cultures for Health,
www.culturesforhealth.com

Herbs and Spices: Mountain Rose Herbs, www.mountainroseherbs.com

Superfoods & More: Ultimate Superfoods, www.ultimatesuperfoods.com

CUSTOM SUPERFOOD ADD-ON GUIDE

This is an easy guide to follow when building your own custom drink or if you'd like to add something extra to one of the recipes in this book.

ACAI POWDER	1 tsp	FRESH GINGER ROOT	1-inch slice
ALMONDS	¼ cup	GOJI BERRIES	1–3 tbsp
ALMOND BUTTER	2 tbsp	HEMP SEEDS	1–2 tbsp
ALMOND EXTRACT	1 tsp	HOLY BASIL EXTRACT	⅛ tsp
ASHWAGANDHA EXTRACT	⅛ tsp	KALE	2–3 large leaves + stems
AVOCADO	¼ cup	LUCUMA	1 tsp–1 tbsp
BRAZIL NUTS	¼ cup	MACA POWDER	1 tsp–1 tbsp
CACAO POWDER	1–3 tbsp	MESQUITE	1 tsp
CACAO NIBS	1–2 tbsp	MORINGA POWDER	1 tsp
CAMU CAMU POWDER	1–2 tsp	PEPPERMINT EXTRACT	½ tsp
CASHEWS	¼ cup	SHILAJIT EXTRACT	⅛ tsp
CEREMONIAL CACAO	1–3 tbsp	SPIRULINA	¼ tsp
CHAGA POWDER	½ tsp	SPINACH	heaping handful
CHAI SPICE	1–2 tsp	TURMERIC PASTE	1 tsp–1 tbsp
CHIA SEEDS	1 tbsp	VANILLA EXTRACT	1 tsp–1 tbsp
CHLORELLA	¼ tsp	WALNUTS	¼ cup
COCONUT OIL	1 tbsp		

NUT + SEED SOAKING GUIDE

While you don't have to soak nuts or seeds at all if you're in a pinch, it is ideal if you have the time and foresight, as the soaking process releases toxins, increases nutrient bioavailability, and makes the mylk more digestible. Refrigerate if soaking for more than two hours. Once they're done soaking, strain out the water (do not save) and gently rinse the nuts or seeds. Always use filtered or spring water when soaking. Not all seeds need to be soaked; see the chart below.

ALMONDS	12	Hours
BRAZIL NUTS	2	Hours
CASHEWS	2	Hours
COCONUT*	0	Hours
FLAX SEEDS	2	Hours
HAZELNUTS	8	Hours
HEMP SEEDS	0	Hours
MACADAMIA NUTS	2	Hours
PECANS	8	Hours
PUMPKIN SEEDS	6	Hours
SUNFLOWER SEEDS	4	Hours
WALNUTS	8	Hours

Coconut mylk can be made using dried coconut, raw coconut meat, or canned coconut. Raw coconut meat usually comes frozen; defrost before use. For canned coconut, use full-fat, BPA-free can (I recommend Native Forest or Thai Kitchen); dilute with water 1:3.

233

INGREDIENT GLOSSARY

ACAI berry comes from the acai palm tree, native to Central and South America. It is high in antioxidants, lowers cholesterol and increases heart health, supports healthy skin, aids digestion, boosts the immune system, improves mental focus, and combats aging.

ACTIVATED CHARCOAL is a powerful substance used to remove toxins (everything from drug or alcohol poisoning to spider bites), reduce bloating, lower cholesterol, whiten teeth, filter water, clear mold, support adrenal glands, and topically for skin health and to heal wounds (poison ivy, spider bites, acne, etc.).

ALMONDS are delicious tree nuts that are filled with healthy fats, antioxidants, fiber, protein, magnesium, manganese, vitamin B2, vitamin E, copper, and phosphorous. They are alkalizing, lower blood pressure and cholesterol, and help to manage healthy weight.

ALOE is a wonderful plant that is most well known for healing and soothing burns. It also provides great benefits for general skin and hair health and can be used internally to support oral health, combat tooth decay, lower cholesterol and blood sugar, and aid digestion. It is high in antioxidants and has tremendous antibacterial and anti-inflammatory properties.

APPLES are the quintessential fruit. They contain important antioxidants, nutrients, and fiber. This common fruit is linked to reducing heart disease, cancer prevention, reducing the risk of diabetes, whitening teeth, reducing cholesterol, protecting against Alzheimer's and Parkinson's, easing digestion, boosting the immune system, preventing cataracts, and detoxifying the liver.

APPLE CIDER VINEGAR offers a great deal of cleansing benefits, including promoting weight loss, whitening teeth, soothing a sore throat, boosting energy, lowering blood sugar, relieving indigestion, and alleviating symptoms of diabetes. It can also be used topically as a hair wash and potent skin cleanser.

ASHWAGANDHA, also known as Indian ginseng, is a root used in Ayurvedic and Traditional Chinese Medicine that is high in antioxidants and boosts the immune system. It is used to fight cancer and diabetes, regulate the thyroid and adrenal glands, increase stamina, relieve stress, reduce inflammation, treat asthma, promote sexual health, and ease arthritis pain.

ASTRAGALUS is a potent adaptogenic root used in Traditional Chinese Medicine as a powerful immune booster. It is used to combat stress and disease, prevent heart and kidney disease, treat colds, relieve symptoms of diabetes and asthma, reduce inflammation, and heal wounds.

AVOCADOS are a deliciously healthy, fatty fruit that has become quite a star in the health food world, and for good reasons. They are rich in monounsaturated fats, lower bad cholesterol and raise good cholesterol. Avocadoes are a great source of vitamin E, boosting immunity and making them beneficial both internally and externally for skin and hair health. They are also high in protein.

BANANAS are ubiquitous in every household and even convenience stores. Predominantly known as a good source of potassium, they also contain fiber, antioxidants, and vitamins C and B6. They are used to ease digestion, stimulate weight loss, increase heart health, and moderate blood sugar levels.

BEE POLLEN is the food of the bees; while I love its benefits, I rarely use it anymore after speaking with our beekeepers, as its powerful medicine needs to be going to the bees that are so dutifully nourishing our planet. It is 40 percent protein, contains a high amount of amino acids, is extremely nutrient dense, and is one of the most nourishing foods known. Sourced carefully and locally, it is a wonderful treatment to seasonal allergies. It is also used to reduce inflammation, boost energy, promote heart health, aid digestion, support a healthy prostate, restore fertility, is an aphrodisiac, and can be used topically for skin health.

BEETS are the candy of the earth. This sweet root vegetable contains high levels of vitamin C, fiber, potassium, manganese, magnesium, iron and folate. Their health benefits include boosting stamina, lowering blood pressure, detoxifying blood and the liver, cancer prevention, and reducing inflammation.

BLUEBERRIES are a popular, everyday household fruit loaded with antioxidants, fiber, potassium, vitamin C, and vitamin B6. They are well known for increasing heart health, lowering cholesterol, boosting brain health, fighting cancer, supporting healthy skin, easing digestion, and assisting weight loss.

BRAZIL NUTS are not only delicious and creamy, but these nuts also contain selenium, protein, iron, calcium, magnesium, potassium, and sodium. They are most well known for stimulating hair growth and improving heart health. They also lower cholesterol, reduce inflammation, support thyroid function, and protect against cancer. Due to their high concentration of selenium, it is important not to consume too many, as too much of this mineral can cause negative side effects.

BURDOCK ROOT is used to purify blood, detoxify the liver, aid in digestion, reduce inflammation, balance hormones, improve skin health, and lower blood pressure.

CARDAMOM is related to ginger and shares many similar healing properties. It is a warming spice used to aid digestion, combat nausea, relieve heartburn, stimulate appetite, and assist elimination of waste from the kidneys.

CARROTS are popular root vegetables filled with beta-carotene, fiber, antioxidants, vitamins A, C, K, and B8, folate, copper, potassium, iron, and manganese. They are known for improving vision, enhancing skin health, preventing cancer, fighting the signs of aging, detoxifying the liver, preventing heart disease and stroke, and promoting oral health.

CASHEWS are packed with vitamins E, K, and B6, as well as copper, phosphorous, zinc, magnesium, iron, selenium, and protein. Their health benefits include relieving migraines, increasing cognitive function, lowering blood pressure, protecting skin health, strengthening bones, and reducing the risk of cancer.

CAYENNE PEPPER is a mighty medicine that is well known for its cleansing properties. It can be used to increase circulation, neutralize acidity, alleviate heartburn, treat gout and paralysis, heal sore throats, combat cold and flu, aid digestion, reduce inflammation, boost metabolism, ease cramps, heal topical wounds, relieve allergies, and prevent migraines.

CELERY is a wonderful source of antioxidants, enzymes, vitamins C, K, and B6, folate, fiber, electrolytes, and potassium. It is an anti-inflammatory that has been shown to lower blood pressure and cholesterol levels, enhance digestion and promote weight loss, reduce the risk of ulcers, prevent dehydration, and improve the liver, skin, and eye health.

CEREMONIAL CACAO is fermented, sun-dried, lightly roasted, and peeled. This is a traditional preparation method of Mayan culture. It has healing benefits similar to raw cacao (see p 246) and can be used to both promote health and for ceremonial purposes.

CHAGA is regarded as the "king of medicinal mushrooms," known by Siberians as the "Gift from God" and the "Mushroom of Immortality." It grows primarily on birch trees in colder climates in the Northern Hemisphere and is very woody, inedible unless decocted into a tea, ground into a fine powder, or extracted in alcohol. We source ours from local wild crafters utilizing sustainable practices. Chaga is used for longevity, immune system support, and digestive support, is extremely high in antioxidants and nutrients, has shown anti-cancer properties, and it is considered the most potent adaptogen.

CHIA seeds are nutritional powerhouses from Central America that contain essential fatty acids, dietary fiber, and are high in antioxidants, vitamins, minerals, and protein. Their fiber and healthy fat content is beneficial to diabetics, as it balances blood sugar levels. They are also known to boost energy and metabolism and are often used by endurance athletes. One ounce of chia seeds contains 18 percent of the recommended daily amount of calcium, making it a great plant-based source of this fundamental mineral known to build and maintain strong bones.

CHLORELLA is a green algae that helps to negate the effects of radiation, lowers blood pressure and cholesterol, detoxifies the body, increases cardiovascular health, and supports healthy hormonal function.

CHERRIES are extremely rich in antioxidants, vitamin E, and vitamin C. They contain melatonin, which promotes restful sleep. They are used to prevent cancer, provide arthritis pain relief, alleviate muscle pain, reduce stomach fat, protect the heart, are anti-inflammatory, and reduce the risk of gout.

CILANTRO is a good source of antioxidants, beta-carotene, vitamins, and fiber. It is most known for its ability to detox heavy metals, but it can also be used to relieve anxiety, lower blood sugar levels, improve sleep, treat diabetes, and ease digestion.

CINNAMON is a highly medicinal and very delicious culinary spice. Go for Ceylon if you can, as Cassia is not true cinnamon and can cause damage with larger doses. Cinnamon is packed with antioxidants, is anti-inflammatory, antifungal, antibacterial, reduces the risk of heart disease, protects against brain disease (such as Alzheimer's and Parkinson's), protects the body from cancer, combats HIV, and regulates the metabolism and blood sugar levels, therefore having an antidiabetic effect.

CLOVES are tiny medicinal powerhouses in the spice world. Used in Ayurvedic medicine, they are antifungal, antibacterial, antiseptic, and analgesic. They are also brimming with antioxidants, manganese, omega-3 fatty acids, fiber, and vitamins. Cloves are used to treat toothaches, reduce inflammation, improve digestion, heal wounds, relieve upper respiratory infections, and as an aphrodisiac to increase sexual vitality.

COCONUT is one of the most magical and versatile fruits in my personal opinion. It is a great source of fiber, vitamins, minerals, and fatty acids. Check out the descriptions for coconut oil and coconut water for more details.

COCONUT AMINOS is aged and salted coconut sap used as a soy-free, gluten-free alternative to tamari or soy sauce that is significantly higher in amino acids.

COCONUT OIL is easily in my top five favorite ingredients. This healthy fat can be used topically to improve skin and hair health and has antibacterial properties that help heal wounds. It is linked to improving memory and brain function, promoting heart health by increasing good cholesterol, aiding in weight loss by supporting a healthy thyroid, and is an anti-inflammatory used to relieve arthritis. This oil has a high heat point, making it great for cooking.

COCONUT WATER is a delicious, refreshing, low-calorie natural beverage perfect for replacing sports drinks for optimal hydration. It is packed with antioxidants, amino acids, enzymes, B-complex vitamins, vitamin C, iron, calcium, potassium, magnesium, manganese, and zinc. With all of this, it lowers blood pressure, boosts the immune system, relieves headaches, promotes weight loss, and supports heart health.

CORIANDER is the seed of Cilantro and shares in its medicinal benefits.

CUCUMBERS are extremely hydrating fruits containing vitamins B1, B5, B7, C, and K, as well as beta-carotene, manganese, copper, and potassium. They reduce the risk of cancer, are anti-inflammatory, protect brain health, decrease stress, aid digestion, promote heart health, help manage weight loss, and reduce bad breath.

DAMIANA is a small shrub with leaves that have been used in Central America for thousands of years for their aphrodisiac properties to enhance sexual potency. It has also been used for cleansing and suppressing appetite.

DANDELION is possibly one of the most wonderful wild gifts that the plant world offers. This invasive species grows abundantly on all continents and is widely considered to be a weed. However, the medicinal properties are immense, and the entire plant is edible (roots, stem, leaves, flower). Dandelion is high in antioxidants, vitamins A, C, K, and B6, along with calcium, iron, potassium, magnesium and manganese, to name a few. Amidst the many benefits, this bitter plant it is known to lower blood sugar, treat AIDS and herpes, fight cancer, support the liver, increase vision, purify blood, ease digestion, and treat anemia, jaundice, and gout. Best of all, you can walk outside and harvest it yourself! Just make sure you harvest away from heavy trafficked roads and on land that is not treated with pesticides.

DATES are one of nature's most magical candies. We use both deglet and medjool; while medjool are more expensive, they are also much more luxurious, caramel-like, and superior for raw desserts. This natural sweetener is better than other alternatives as it helps to stabilize blood sugar levels. Beyond the sweet factor, dates also contain three times the potassium of bananas, and are great sources of manganese and magnesium, along with many other vitamins and minerals, such as calcium, iron, phosphorous, sodium, and zinc. They are also aphrodisiacs, known to increase your sexual stamina!

ELDERBERRY is an extremely valuable addition to any medicine cabinet. This berry is said to be more effective than the flu shot in preventing colds and flu. It is a well-known antibacterial and antiviral that is high in antioxidants, used to lower cholesterol, improve eyesight, boost immunity, alleviate coughs, and support heart health.

FENNEL is a good source of vitamins C and B6, iron, calcium, fiber, and potassium, to name a few. It is known for lowering cholesterol and therefore decreasing the risk of heart disease. Fennel is also well known for easing digestion, relieving anemia, treating colic, and regulating menstrual disorders.

GARLIC, while widely used in the kitchen, has long been used for its tremendous medicinal properties. It contains good amounts of antioxidants, manganese, calcium, fiber, selenium, vitamins B6, C, and B1, potassium, iron, copper, and phosphorous. Garlic is used to boost the immune system, combat illness, lower blood pressure, increase good cholesterol, prevent against Alzheimer's and dementia, extend longevity, detoxify heavy metals, enhance athletic ability, and improve bone health.

GINGER is a popular spicy root that has long been used for easing digestive issues like nausea, appetite loss, pain, and motion sickness. It is also known as an anti-inflammatory to reduce muscle pain, lower blood sugar levels, reduce menstrual pain, lower cholesterol, prevent cancer, improve cognitive function, and fight infections.

GINSENG is a powerful root used in Traditional Chinese Medicine to boost energy, reduce stress, lower blood sugar and cholesterol, treat diabetes, and restore male sexual function.

GOJI BERRIES are high in vitamin C and fiber and are known to boost the immune system, increase focus, lower blood pressure, ease inflammation, promote healthy skin, and protect the eyes, among a long list of other benefits.

GOTU KOLA is an herb originating from Asia that has been used in India, China, and Africa for thousands of years. It is used to promote restful sleep, alleviate fatigue, purify blood, safeguard the heart, ease anxiety and depression, accelerate wound healing, enhance skin health, promote circulation, and improve memory.

HABANERO PEPPERS are the hottest of all commercially grown peppers. They contain high concentrations of vitamins A and C, fiber and capsaicin. They are linked to reducing cancer growth, decreasing inflammation, increasing cardiovascular health, and preventing diabetes.

HEMP SEEDS are insanely powerful nutritional superheroes! They are filled with omega-3 and omega-6 fatty acids, rich in protein and healthy fats, and a good source of vitamin E, phosphorous, potassium, sodium, magnesium, sulfur, calcium, iron, and zinc. Hemp seeds are used to reduce the risk of heart disease, support skin health, relieve symptoms of menopause and PMS, and aid digestion.

HOLY BASIL, also known as *Tulsi*, Sanskrit for "the incomparable one," is regarded in Ayurveda as an "elixir of life," known to promote longevity. It can be used to care for oral health, relieve stress and muscle pain, reduce inflammation, support the respiratory system, and treat fever, asthma, and heart disease.

HORSERADISH is a root vegetable that's a good source of fiber, vitamin C, folate, zinc, manganese, potassium, calcium and magnesium. This root is known to fight infection, prolong life, fight cancer, heal sinusitis and urinary tract infections, treat dandruff, protect the human body from toxic chemicals, stimulate blood flow, and relieve muscle and arthritic pain.

HORSETAIL is an herb high in silica that is used to strengthen bones, hair, and nails, and to enhance cognitive function, relieve bronchitis, and more. It is also anti-inflammatory and antifungal.

KALE is one of my favorite dark leafy greens. It is high in antioxidants, fiber, iron, vitamins A, C, and K, protein, folate, and magnesium. It is good for detoxing and supporting the liver, reduces inflammation, and lowers cholesterol.

KAVA KAVA is a sacred root originating in Polynesia. It is well known as a powerful nervine that is used to relieve stress, anxiety, and muscle pain, as well as to support restful sleep.

LEMONS contain citric acid, vitamin C, B-complex, calcium, copper, iron, magnesium, phosphorous, potassium, and fiber. This common citrus is known to lower the risk of stroke, prevent asthma, aid in digestion and detoxification, promotes healthy skin, enhances weight loss, and boosts energy and mood.

LEMON BALM is a wonderfully cooling, calming herb known to reduce stress and anxiety, promote sleep, increase appetite, and ease digestive pain.

LIME is a delicious citrus with high amounts of vitamin C and many health benefits, such as weight loss, enhanced digestion, increased eye care, improving oral health, relieving diabetes and lowering blood sugar, lowering cholesterol, protecting the heart, easing arthritis pain, reducing fevers, preventing gout, aiding weight loss, healing urinary disorders, and more.

LUCUMA is a fruit from South America (primarily Peru) that is mostly found in northern climates as a dried powder. It is used as a natural sweetener and is a popular ice cream flavor in Peru. This delicious superfood contains beta-carotene, iron, zinc, vitamin B3, calcium, and protein.

MACA is a deliciously sweet and slightly malty root vegetable that grows in the high Andes of Peru and has long been used for its potent medicinal benefits. Maca is a safe adaptogen that is rich in vitamins B, C, and E and provides a good dosage of amino acids, calcium, zinc, magnesium, iron, and phosphorous. It is also used as an aphrodisiac to increase libido and endurance. This is a superfood that I like to take occasional short breaks from, as it may become ineffective with long-term consistent use; when I return to using it regularly, I feel the benefits much more. Due to its increase in popularity and the research on its many health benefits, this plant has recently become highly sought after, with prices increasing from Chinese brokers. Be careful where you source this superfood, as it may soon be contaminated with filler ingredients or genetically modified.

MANGO is a deliciously alkalizing tropical fruit that is high in vitamins A, B6, C, and K, as well as iron, potassium, and calcium. Mangoes lower cholesterol, fight cancer, promote weight loss, regulate diabetes, ease digestion, boost the immune system, increase cognitive function, and enhance skin health.

MAPLE SYRUP is made from the sap of maple trees. Beyond being insanely delicious, this sweetener contains antioxidants, zinc, manganese, calcium, and potassium, is anti-inflammatory and has a lower glycemic index than raw cane sugar, making it a better alternative as it helps to regulate blood sugar levels. Make sure you're buying *pure* maple syrup, not the fake maple-flavored stuff filled with high fructose corn syrup.

MATCHA GREEN TEA is jam-packed with high doses of antioxidants, enhances memory and concentration, burns calories, supports heart health, detoxifies the body, boosts immunity, increases energy and endurance, and provides calming effects.

MESQUITE is a leguminous staple food that has been used by Native Americans for thousands of years. It is high in protein, used as a paleo / raw flour, and contains good amounts of calcium, magnesium, iron, potassium, zinc, and the amino acid lysine. It has a slightly sweet, nutty flavor and is very low on the glycemic index scale, making it a safe sweetener alternative.

MORINGA leaf powder is a magical green superfood that is easily grown and very sustainable. The seeds and roots are also used medicinally and for water purifying benefits. It provides significant amounts of protein, calcium, potassium, and vitamins A, C, and E. This powerful plant also delivers a good source of antioxidants, fights inflammation, relieves some symptoms of diabetes, supports brain health, protects the liver and cardiovascular health, and shows antifungal and antibacterial benefits that are beneficial to healing wounds, blood and urinary tract infections, and digestive issues.

NETTLE is a safe and extremely nourishing, supportive, adaptogenic herb. It has an extensive list of benefits including being used to ease joint paint and arthritis, support urinary issues, clear eczema, stop internal and external bleeding, purify the blood, relieve congestion, reduce inflammation, boost immunity, support oral health, and promote thyroid health.

NUTMEG is a popular culinary spice with many medicinal benefits including aiding sleep, boosting immunity, clearing skin, enhancing digestion, promoting oral health, relieving joint and muscle pain, promoting blood circulation and a healthy liver, and increasing cognitive function. It is also antibacterial and is a good source of potassium, calcium, manganese, and iron.

NUTRITIONAL YEAST (commonly known as "nooch") is typically grown on sugar beets or molasses; I look for the latter, as sugar beets are predominantly genetically engineered. Nutritional yeast is a complete source of protein and vitamins, is high in fiber, and contains folates, thiamine, selenium, zinc, riboflavin, and niacin. While it does not naturally contain vitamin B12, it is often added in. It increases energy and has antiviral, antibacterial, and immune-boosting qualities. This inactive yeast is generally considered safe in regards to concern about yeast overgrowth or infection.

OAT STRAW is a deeply nourishing herb used for promoting longevity, restoring the nervous system, reducing stress, supporting heart health and cholesterol, balancing emotions, treating skin problems, and enhancing sexual vitality. It is high in calcium, protein, silica, and B vitamins.

OREGANO is a household culinary herb that has powerful medicinal benefits, especially in its concentrated essential oil. It is high in antioxidants and rich in fiber, iron, manganese, calcium, vitamin E, and omega-3 and omega-6 fatty acids. It can be used to treat skin conditions, boost the immune system, reduce inflammation, treat intestinal parasites, alleviate upper respiratory infections, relieve headaches and allergies, ease menstrual cramps and muscle pain, clear acne, and so much more. It is a known antiviral, antifungal, and antibacterial, and also beneficial in treating candida overgrowth.

PARSLEY is a wonderful source of vitamins K, C, E, B6, B12, and A, as well as iron, calcium, magnesium, manganese, potassium, zinc, phosphorous, and copper. It is used to promote bone health and prevent both diabetes and cancer.

PASSIONFLOWER is a sedative plant used in herbal medicine to reduce anxiety, relieve insomnia, and soothe stomach pain.

PEPPERMINT is a popular antimicrobial herb enjoyed for both its cooling and calming benefits. It is also used to ease anxiety, digestion, menstrual cramps, muscle and nerve pain, and irritable bowel syndrome. While peppermint is a relaxant, it is simultaneously a stimulant used to increase energy and alertness; avoid using before sleep.

PINEAPPLE is a delicious tropical fruit containing good amounts of vitamin C, vitamin B6, beta-carotene, calcium, magnesium, folate, manganese, potassium, and copper. It is also known to contain high amounts of bromelain. Bromelain is a naturally occurring, plant-based digestive enzyme used to reduce inflammation, ease arthritis and joint pain, boost immunity, and more. Pineapple can also be used to promote skin health, prevent cancer, fight colds and flu, strengthen bones, benefit oral health and vision, and increase circulation.

PUMPKIN SEEDS contain magnesium, zinc, omega-3 and omega-6 fatty acids, fiber, and antioxidants. Their health benefits include increasing heart health, boosting immunity, improving prostate health, decreasing the effects of diabetes, alleviating menopausal symptoms, promoting restful sleep, and reducing inflammation.

RASPBERRIES are scrumptious little berries containing strong antioxidants, vitamins C, K, and E, fiber, manganese, magnesium, omega-3 fatty acids, quercetin and gallic acid. They fight cancer, heart and circulatory disease, are anti-inflammatory, improve skin health, promote weight loss, support female health, and boost the immune system.

RAW CACAO is the pure, unprocessed form of the well-known cocoa or chocolate. It is packed with powerful antioxidants, as well as many vitamins and minerals such as magnesium, calcium, zinc, sulfur, iron, manganese, potassium, and vitamins B1, B2, B3, B5, B9, C and E. Cacao is used as a mood enhancer, aphrodisiac, and hormone balancer. Raw cacao also helps to prevent heart disease, resets metabolism, improves skin health, increases cognitive function, aids digestion, and provides the body with healthy fats. While it does boost energy, it does not actually contain caffeine, but a similar extract.

RAW CACAO BUTTER is the fat extracted from raw cacao beans.

RAW CACAO NIBS are simply broken down bits of cacao beans.

RAW CACAO POWDER is processed by cold-pressing cacao beans and removing the fat.

RAW HONEY is a magical, sweet gift made by bees foraging nectar from flowers. A lot of honey is now produced unnaturally on a massive scale, shipping bees across the country to pollinate large, genetically engineered monoculture farms and feeding them high fructose syrup sugar water, and using other chemicals in this highly unsustainable practice. We owe endless gratitude to the beekeepers who are committed to the ancient, sacred practice of taking care of our beloved bees, who play a crucial role in maintaining the food supply that we depend upon. Local raw honey (and other bee products such as pollen and propolis) provides profound health benefits, such as allergy relief, and contains powerful antioxidants, 22 amino acids, 27 minerals, and 5,000 enzymes! It also contains antibacterial and antiviral properties, known to heal wounds topically and deliver wonderful healing benefits internally.

RED CLOVER is a readily available wild edible and medicinal plant that you can find right outside your front door. It has been used for cancer prevention and to reduce high cholesterol, aid in digestion, and to treat whooping cough, common cough, asthma, bronchitis, and sexually transmitted diseases. Many women use it to alleviate symptoms of menopause and PMS.

REISHI are more readily abundant and sustainable than chaga, as they regenerate every year instead of taking several decades to grow. This medicinal mushroom is an adaptogen used to boost the immune system, relieve anxiety, lower blood pressure and high cholesterol, alleviate bronchitis, insomnia, and asthma, and has been used to treat kidney disease, cancer, and liver disease.

ROMAINE LETTUCE is a good source of fiber, manganese, potassium, copper, iron, biotin, and vitamins B1 and C. It increases heart health, decreases bad cholesterol, and lowers blood pressure.

ROSE PETALS act as an aphrodisiac, aid in weight loss, relieve stress and depression, and promote healthy skin.

ROSEMARY is a medicinal culinary herb with antifungal, antibacterial, antiseptic, and anti-inflammatory properties. It is used to relieve headaches, improve memory, enhance mood, reduce pain, and help to fight cancer.

SCHISANDRA is known as the "five-flavor berry" in Traditional Chinese Medicine, as it contains all five flavors: sweet, sour, bitter, pungent, and astringent. It is an adaptogenic berry high in antioxidants used to promote longevity and overall vitality. Schisandra is known to support the liver, fight adrenal fatigue, lower inflammation, improve digestion, increase mental clarity, boost energy, protect the skin, enhance hormonal health, and increase libido.

SHILAJIT is an organic mineral pitch known as the "rock of life" from the terrain of the Himalayas. It is considered the root of Ayurvedic medicine. Taken alone, this herb will strengthen the immune system, fortify cells and muscles, and can be used as an anti-oxidant, an anti-stressor, anti-allergen, and antiasthmatic. When used with any other Ayurvedic herb it is considered to boost the health effects of both. It is also historically believed to increase longevity and have nutritional, cleansing, and detoxifying properties. Storage tip: do not refrigerate or leave in a cool, moist space, as shilajit will turn to a still useable, yet rocky, gooey substance.

SKULLCAP is a powerful plant used in Traditional Chinese Medicine to relieve anxiety and stabilize moods, offer pain relief, support the nervous system, promote liver health, manage diabetes, lower cholesterol, aid in weight loss, and prevent cancer.

SPIRULINA is cyanobacteria that is considered to be one of the most potent foods on the planet! Spirulina detoxifies heavy metals, eliminates candida, lowers blood pressure, improves cholesterol, boosts energy and endurance, alleviates allergies and sinus issues, speeds weight loss, prevents cancer, and so much more! It is high in antioxidants and chlorophyll, rich in protein, and is a good source of vitamins A, B1, B2, B3, B6, B9, C, D and E, as well as calcium (26 times that of milk), potassium, chromium, copper, magnesium, manganese, phosphorous, sodium, selenium, and zinc. It is also a highly absorbable source of iron.

SEAWEEDS (Arame, Wakame, Nori, Dulse, Kombu, etc.) are high in protein and minerals such as iodine, calcium, iron, and magnesium. They provide more vitamin C than oranges and contain antiviral, antibacterial and anti-inflammatory properties. Seaweed helps to maintain healthy thyroid function, which has many benefits including reducing fatigue and high cholesterol, balancing hormones, and increasing muscle strength.

SPINACH is a powerful green that is a good source of protein, iron, calcium, potassium, manganese, magnesium, copper, fiber, zinc, choline, and vitamins A, B1, B2, B6, C, E, and K. Its health benefits include managing diabetes, preventing cancer and asthma, supporting healthy digestion, enhancing skin and hair health, increasing bone health, and lowering blood pressure.

STEVIA is a sweetener and sugar substitute made from the leaves of the stevia plant, something you can easily grow in your backyard or window garden. Stevia has zero calories and is 200 times sweeter than sugar; be careful, a little goes a long way!

STRAWBERRIES provide a great source of vitamins C and B6, antioxidants, manganese, magnesium, potassium, copper, and omega-3 fatty acids. These delicious berries boost immunity, promote eye health, regulate blood pressure, reduce bad cholesterol and inflammation, enhance skin health, fight cancer, and support weight management.

SUNFLOWER SEEDS are filled with vitamin E, B vitamins, copper, folate, niacin, thiamin, phosphorous, selenium, and essential fatty acids. These small seeds reduce the risk of cardiovascular disease, promote healthy cholesterol levels, support thyroid health, enhance mood, protect the heart, and relieve symptoms of PMS.

SWEET POTATOES are an excellent source of vitamins A, C, B1, B2, B6, and D, along with manganese, phosphorous, potassium, fiber, and copper. Their health benefits include reducing heart disease, promoting healthy skin, boosting immunity, strengthening bones, relieving anxiety, regulating blood sugar levels, and protecting against cancer.

THYME is a standard household culinary herb with great medicinal value. It has one of the most potent levels of antioxidants among herbs, is extremely rich in potassium, iron, calcium, manganese, magnesium, selenium, beta-carotene, and vitamins A, B-complex, C, E, and K. It is used to relieve whooping cough, sore throat, bronchitis, stomachaches, arthritis, and more.

TURMERIC ROOT is a rhizomatous, herbaceous perennial plant of the ginger family indigenous to southwest India that's used fresh or dried as a powder. Most known for the active ingredient curcumin, turmeric has been used in Ayurvedic and Traditional Chinese Medicine for thousands of years with a wide range of benefits. It acts as an anti-inflammatory, antioxidant, antitumor, antibacterial, and antiviral. Consuming with both black pepper and healthy fats (i.e., coconut mylk, coconut oil, nut or seed butters, etc.) tremendously enhances its bioavailability in the body, which increases the profound positive medicinal benefits it has to offer.

VANILLA is a popular flavor that has tremendous health benefits as a good source of magnesium, calcium, potassium, and manganese. These minerals are beneficial to stabalize moods, promote metabolism, support the nervous system, reduce stress and anxiety, regulate blood pressure levels, balance electrolytes, increase heart health, and relieve symptoms of PMS. It is also a known aphrodisiac.

WALNUTS are extremely rich in polyunsaturated fats, primarily omega-3 and omega-6 fatty acids. They're also a good source of antioxidants, protein, manganese, and copper. Walnuts are used to fight prostate and breast cancer, improve heart health, manage weight, improve male reproductive health, boost cognitive function, and reduce symptoms of diabetes.

WHEATGRASS is a powerful superfood, providing the best-known source of living chlorophyll. Liquid chlorophyll is able to penetrate cell walls to heal and renew, being a major asset to the anti-aging process. This super green is high in magnesium, rich in protein, contains vitamins A, B-complex, C, E, and K, and 17 amino acids. It is used to purify the liver, cleanse blood, remove toxins, lower blood sugar, combat tooth decay, relieve a sore throat, improve digestion, and increase energy and endurance. It can also be used topically to ease arthritis, sooth itching, and clear skin.

RESOURCES

BOOKS:

The Body Ecology Diet: Recovering Your Health and Rebuilding Your Immunity, by Donna Gates and Linda Schatz. This book explores the links of chronic health issues with poor digestive health and fungal / yeast infections. Gates focuses on building a healthy gut by looking at acidic versus alkaline foods and how turning to an alkaline diet filled with probiotics and mineral-rich foods, such as seaweeds, can transform your health.

The China Study: Startling Implications for Diet, Weight Loss and Long-term Health, by T. Colin Campbell, PhD and Thomas M. Campbell, MD. This book reviews the relationship between consumption of animal protein and chronic disease, such as diabetes and heart disease, concluding that a whole foods, plant-based diet can prevent and reverse these Western diseases.

Wheat Belly: Lose the Wheat, Lose the Weight, and Find Your Path Back to Health, by William Davis, MD. *Wheat Belly* digs into the adverse health effects of wheat consumption, especially what is on the market and added to so many food products today. Whether you have celiac disease, are wheat intolerant, suffer from non-celiac gluten sensitivity, or are just looking to improve your health, Davis provides a guide to wheat-free living.

The Wheatgrass Book, by Ann Wigmore, dives into the healthful world of wheatgrass—nutrition, growing, juicing—and its many uses. I call this "The Wheatgrass Bible," as it is jam packed with everything you need to know about it. Wigmore, founder of the Hippocrates Health Institute, made this amazing super green popular decades ago!

DOCUMENTARIES:

Fat, Sick and Nearly Dead follows the cross-country journey of Australian Joe Cross on his 60-day juice fast under the care of Dr. Joel Fuhrman. On his journey, Joe meets and inspires Phil Staples, an obese trucker who happens to have the same rare disease that Joe cures himself of, to try out juice fasting.

Fed Up looks at the obesity epidemic and dives into our corrupt food system, with a focus on processed foods and Big Sugar lobbyists.

Forks Over Knives reviews the work of Dr. T. Colin Campbell and Dr. Caldwell Esselstyn. Their studies show that many affluent diseases, such as cancer and cardiovascular disease, can be prevented and reversed with a whole foods, plant-based diet that eliminates processed foods and animal protein.

The Gerson Miracle shares the life work of Dr. Max Gerson of The Gerson Therapy, a method based on a whole foods, plant-based diet that is shown to heal a variety of chronic Western diseases.

May I Be Frank covers the forty-two-day cleanse of fifty-four-year-old Frank Ferrante who works alongside the Café Gratitude team on his transformational journey to weight loss, healing himself of hepatitis C, releasing unhealthy habits, and finding love.

WEBSITES:

Dr. Aviva Romm, doctor, midwife, herbalist, author, www.avivaromm.com

Dr. Mark Hyman, author and founder and medical director of the UltraWellness Center, www.drhyman.com

Dr. T. Colin Campbell, professor emeritus of nutritional biochemistry at Cornell University, author, founder of T. Colin Campbell Center for Nutrition Studies, www.nutritionstudies.org

Dr. Caldwell Esselstyn, director of the cardiovascular prevention and reversal program at the Cleveland Clinic Wellness Institute, surgeon, author, www.dresselstyn.com

Dr. Joel Fuhrman, Nutrition Research Foundation's director of research, author, www.drfuhrman.com

Free Fire Cider, www.freefirecider.com, was created by herbalists working with Rosemary Gladstar to fight the Tradition, Not Trademark battle against Shire City Herbals. Shire City Herbals trademarked this traditional remedy in 2014 and has been pursuing lawsuits against other herbalists, small and large, who use this name. This organization is working to protect common herbal terms and keep them in the public domain.

ACKNOWLEDGMENTS

The biggest thank-you goes to my amazing parents, who have been beyond supportive of my life journey; they are the reason I am who I am and have felt safe following my heart and my passions. They raised me on good healthy food and supported me through the extremely difficult struggles of being a restaurant owner. To my brother, Jonathan, for being my first role model, an inspiration, and such a strong, ever-present support.

I also have so much gratitude for Desha Peacock, my business and lifestyle coach and friend, who connected me with Skyhorse and helped me to realize my dream of publishing my first cookbook and has supported me throughout the process. Wyatt Andrews for his stellar photography work and friendship. Noelle VanHendrick for showing me the most beautifully grounded and humble practice of love and light through her life and gorgeous work; I had the honor of borrowing boxes full of Zpots pottery to use in the photographs for this book. Tara Dente, my beautiful friend and housemate, who helped me through one of the hardest times of my life—finishing this book while being immobile with a foot injury for more than three months. Danielle Sessler for her steadfast friendship and encouragement. Marian Flaxman for helping to inspire and break barriers to a very strange and delicious creative culinary fire. Jacob Roberts for helping to inspire and build Superfresh! Molly Lord for guiding me through my dietary triggers early on. Jennifer Esposito for embodying strength through the darkest hours and offering immense support. Jeff Stamler for offering such valuable feedback and constant support.

My incredible Superfresh! crew for helping to make a good handful of the drink recipes during photo shoots, holding down the shop while I was finishing up the manuscript, photos, and then out of commission for months. Eden Love for helping to develop and inspire the original Superfresh! menu. Grace Nolan for standing with Superfresh! since year one in our first location. The community in and around Brattleboro, Vermont, which has supported me and Superfresh! since fall 2012. To our farmers and beekeepers who work so hard to provide us with good food and steward our precious earth.

To my beloved Ithaca family, between Ithaca College, GreenStar, the Factor, and every other inch, for being my first home away from home where I was able to spread my wings and explore my passions (and dietary restrictions) with such great support in a loving community. These years were critical to so much of my current existence, filled with endless nights of cooking, philosophizing, visiting lectures, pouring through endless nutrition literature, and more with the most wonderful friends. It is here that my food journey blossomed and grew like fire, and where I first stumbled upon *The China Study*, which changed so much of my life path. CW for years of friendship, tremendous support, introduction to *The China Study*, and endless intellectual and creative stimulation. Doug Krisch for opening my eyes to the magical medicinal ways of the bees. To Brooke Hansen and Jack Rossen for inspiring me to venture down my path studying food as medicine and paleoethnobotany.

The gratitude I have cannot be contained in these brief acknowledgements; it belongs to everyone whom I have ever been fortunate enough to cross paths with, every experience I have lived, each lesson I have learned and am continuing to process, and to all of the unknown blessings on the way.

ABOUT THE AUTHOR

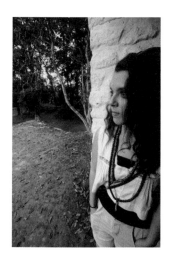

Jessica Jean Weston is owner and executive chef at Superfresh! Organic Café. Jessica studied medical anthropology at Ithaca College and is a certified holistic health coach (Institute for Integrative Nutrition). Jessica has spent her career exploring the broad subject of food as medicine. This professional concentration has led her to work alongside traditional Mayan bush doctors in the forests of Belize, to labor on CSA farms in the Finger Lakes and Green Mountains, to study herbalism, shiatsu, and shamanism in southern Vermont, to provide marketing and outreach coordination at the GreenStar Cooperative Market, and to volunteer at the Ithaca Free Clinic.

Jessica's personal journey to health, navigating a series of food intolerances, as well as discovering what made her feel most vibrant, led her to a non-GMO, plant-based diet free of soy, gluten, dairy, eggs, and meat. Recognizing that everyone has their own path to explore with different physical, emotional, and environmental needs, her goal is to simply share her experiences and knowledge through creating delicious, approachable cuisine, with understanding that no two beings are alike.

Her passion for food runs deep through her Italian roots and endless layers of her life travels, studies, and experiences, and can be seen in the creation of her restaurant in Brattleboro, Vermont. She has a healthy addiction to crafting creative combinations and alternative twists on classic favorites, while aiming to fuel the body, mind, and spirit with the best ingredients possible, and the love for her craft surely seeps through every aspect of her work.

INDEX